MW01227256

PRAISE FOR HANK IN MY HEAD

Hank in My Head is a must-read for anyone seeking inspiration and a deeper understanding of the realities of living with IIH. It is a poignant reminder of the strength that lies within us all and the extraordinary lengths to which we can go for the ones we love. This is a "tear-jerker" warning, but your heart and cup will runneth over!

— VANESSA PENNOYER, PRESIDENT NAWBO KENTUCKY

Knowing Bridgette gives me inspiration. She makes me want to be a better person. The strength and courage I have watched her use to battle against IIH is remarkable. When most would break, she faces it head-on with grace and determination, not allowing it to define her. IIH is a rare disease, one which most people are not familiar with. This book is a perfect gateway to finding answers to questions surrounding IIH, as experienced by someone living with it.

— IRENE PECK, NURSE SCPS

From the moment I met Bridgette, I sensed she was a strong, determined young woman with a huge heart for helping people. In *Hank in My Head*, Bridgette not only validates these impressions but also reveals a profound courage. This book highlights Bridgette's strengths, showcased in a touching vulnerability as she shares her deeply personal account of living with IIH.

— JANA MILLER, CPA

As one who has experienced pain and anguish due to IIH, I was immediately captured by the word pictures that Bridgette Finley has eloquently penned on paper regarding her personal highs and lows that are difficult to express when brain function is not working like it should. I have known Bridgette for years now and to see the Hand of God bring her through deep, difficult times is a testament to God's help and her diligent faith.

— DR. MARK F. HORSTEMEYER, LIBERTY UNIVERSITY SCHOOL OF ENGINEERING DEAN

All of us suffering with the overwhelming and exhausting realities of life with a chronic illness can find encouragement within these pages. Bridgette shares her own raw journey with a heavy dose of vulnerability, bringing hope and even companionship to the reader. Giving a voice to the daily struggles of chronic illness is a gift to those who feel alone in their suffering. Bridgette shares her warrior spirit with her readers in such a beautiful and powerful way.

— SHANNON CARROLL, REGISTERED NURSE, AUTHOR AND SPEAKER

I first met Bridgette when she was a teenager. It was readily apparent that she was much more mature than other kids her age. I suspect this was at least partly due to her journey with multiple unexplained symptoms and learning to cope with them and continue living her life. I am very impressed, though not surprised, that Bridgette has chosen to share her personal story, with the only goal in mind being to help others.

— DAYNA S. EARLY, MD, PROFESSOR OF MEDICINE, DIRECTOR, ENDOSCOPY

HANK IN MY HEAD

EMBRACING LIFE THROUGH OVERCOMING THE CHALLENGES OF IIH

BRIDGETTE FINLEY

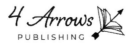

4 Arrows
PUBLISHING

To my beloved husband Bobby, your endless patience, strength, and love have been my anchor through every challenge.

To my wonderful children, McKenzie, Addison, and Ashton, your unwavering support and joy are my greatest treasures.

And to my IIH community, your courage and solidarity have been a beacon of hope and inspiration. This book is a testament to our shared journey and the strength we find in each other.

FOREWORD
DR. STUART YOUNG, OD, FCOVD

My journey alongside Bridgette as she confronts the challenges of idiopathic intracranial hypertension (IIH) began unexpectedly in a local coffee shop. It was during a meeting with her husband that I learned of the details surrounding a social media post she had made detailing nearly nine months of chronic symptoms without relief or diagnosis. She had shared her frustration that she could not get any relief or answers.

After the meeting was over, her husband and I were walking out of the coffee shop to our cars; I offhandedly asked what was going on and inquired about the symptoms she had mentioned in her post. Having been her optometrist for years, her symptoms did not seem to be vision related. She had a chronic "whooshing" or "heartbeat" noise in her ear and was suffering from chronic headaches, two very classic symptoms of IIH.

I asked him how long it had been since she'd had her eyes checked. We scheduled her to come in for an eye exam, even though none of her symptoms seemed visual in nature. At her exam, we discovered that she had papilledema (swollen optic nerves), which is a classic sign of IIH. We were able to quickly make the necessary referrals and get her the help she needed. A lack of treatment of the condition can cause atrophy of the optic nerve and will lead to blindness.

Living with IIH (previously called pseudotumor cerebri) is not easy. It can seem like a continual merry-go-round of odd symptoms and headaches, followed by headaches, and then followed by more headaches. It can be very difficult to explain to doctors how it feels. Often there are no clinical signs, especially at the beginning, to help doctors determine the diagnosis. It can be a frustrating and lonely road.

I've had the good fortune of being acquainted with Bridgette for many years and have always been impressed with her desire and ability to go "all in" with whatever she does. She is "all in" in her piano studio; she is "all in" on the nonprofits that she starts and runs; she is also "all in" on her love of God. Bridgette never does anything halfway. I'm grateful that she has chosen to be "all in" as she tells her story. I'm grateful that she has been humble enough to be open about what it is like to live with this disease. She is compassionate, thorough, and engaging.

In her narrative, Bridgette seamlessly blends personal experience with diligent research into the medical intricacies of IIH. This book is a treasure trove of information for those interested in learning more. This is not just a book that inspires but can serve as a "how to" guide in navigating the medical community in a search for answers.

DISCLAIMER

The content of this book reflects the author's personal opinions and experiences related to idiopathic intracranial hypertension (IIH). It is not intended to serve as medical advice, diagnosis, or treatment. Always seek the guidance of a qualified healthcare professional with any questions you may have regarding a medical condition or treatment. The author and publisher disclaim any responsibility for actions taken based on the information presented in this book.

CONTENTS

Hank in My Head: Embracing Life Through Overcoming the Challenges of IIH

Copyright © 2024 by Bridgette Finley
Published by 4 Arrows Publishing (Kentucky)

All rights reserved. No portion of this book may be reproduced in any form or by electronic or mechanical means, including information storage and retrieval systems, without written permission of the author, except for the use of brief quotations in a book review.

Cover by Madelyn Copperwaite, MC Creative LLC
Cover Artwork by McKenzie Finley, Art by Kenzie
Editing by Jennifer Crosswhite, Tandem Services Ink
Layout by Stephanie Feger, emPower PR Group

First edition, October 2024
ISBN: 979-8-9910474-0-1
Library of Congress Control Number: 2024915532
Created in the United States of America

Scripture quotations marked (NLT) are from The Holy Bible, New Living Translation, Copyright © 1996, 2004, 2015 by Tyndale House Foundation. Used by permission of Tyndale House Publishers, Carol Stream, Illinois 60188. All rights reserved.

Learn more about Bridgette Finley by visiting bridgettefinley.com. Special discounts are available on quantity book purchases.

LETTER TO THE READER

As I sit down to write these words, I am filled with a sense of both nervousness and excitement. Nervousness, because I am about to embark on the vulnerable journey of sharing a deeply personal story. Excitement, because I have the privilege of inviting you into the inner workings of my head, where Hank resides.

Hank in My Head is more than just a book; it's a testament to the resilience of the human spirit and the complexities of living with IIH. In these pages, you'll find raw honesty, moments of clarity, and perhaps a few unexpected revelations. My hope is that this book can help you not just survive, but thrive as you learn to live with debilitating challenges.

Whether you are personally familiar with IIH or encountering it for the first time, my hope is that this book serves as a beacon of understanding and empathy. Through Hank's narrative, I aim to shed light on the often misunderstood realities of this condition and the profound impact it can have on one's life so that you can live more fully.

Have you ever endured relentless head pain, accompanied by a persistent sensation of pressure behind your eyes? Your head and neck stiffen, sending waves of discomfort down your spine. Vision fades into blackouts, while eye floaters dance in your field of view. Optic nerves bear the burden of increased pressure, casting shadows on your sight. Balance becomes difficult; dizziness is a frequent companion. Muscles twitch uncontrollably, adding to the long list of symptoms. Brain fog descends, stealing thoughts and words, making speech a challenge. Even mundane actions like sneezing or bending over provoke disturbance in your head and eyes. Dehydration intensifies the discomfort, while chest and joint pain add to the burden. Nausea becomes a constant presence, disrupting daily life. Sleep eludes you, replaced by a persistent fatigue that weighs heavily on your limbs. Bruises appear without explanation, and spinal fluid leaks from the nose, eyes, and ears. Motor skills falter, leading to instances of dropped objects.

Does any of this sound familiar? Have you had moments of questioning these very symptoms? It is my hope that the pages of this book can encourage you if you're living in the daily battle of IIH.

You might be in a phase of trying to figure out the diagnosis. Maybe lost in the vast sea of doctors, testing, confusion, and frustration of no answers as to why you feel the way you do. Possibly, you are recently diagnosed and excited to finally have an answer as to why you have struggled for so long, yet fearful and anxious as to what the future holds. You might be looking at surgery or facing the prognosis of no cure or fix to your symptoms. Possibly, you are a veteran at living with your illness and you're picking up this book to encourage you to keep pushing forward.

Whatever your reason, dear reader, I invite you to journey alongside me as we navigate the twists and turns of Hank's world. Together, let us explore the depths of life's experience while living with IIH and discover the resilience that lies within us all.

PART ONE
DISCOVERING HANK: THE JOURNEY TO A DIAGNOSIS

I

UNRAVELING THE MYSTERY

"God is our refuge and strength, always ready to help in times of trouble."

— PSALM 46:1 (NLT)

What do you do when life as you know it disappears and you're simply left to figure out how to live again? I vividly recall specific moments throughout my life and wonder why the doctors could not figure out what was wrong with me. Was I going crazy? Was I imagining all the extreme symptoms I knew that I felt? From a young child, I had gone from doctor to doctor attempting to track down symptoms that seemed to have no connection to one another, along with no root cause. I was dismissed time and again because they couldn't find anything wrong with me.

Do you find yourself in this position? Let me tell you that you are not alone. So many of us living with chronic illness have walked this same road to attaining a diagnosis. Navigating the path of knowing something is seriously wrong with your health, but facing constant doctors who cannot pinpoint the issue is a profound challenge. Living with an undiagnosed chronic illness is a complex and often exhausting experience.

THERE IS A ROLLER COASTER OF EMOTIONS ASSOCIATED WITH LIVING WITH AN UNDIAGNOSED CONDITION.

Frustration can arise quickly when you are dealing with persistent symptoms without a clear explanation. It can feel like being trapped in a cycle of seeking answers, but not finding any. At one point in high school, I had to be taken by ambulance when the lights in Dairy Queen had bothered my eyes so much that I passed out. I woke up in the ER to a doctor running a drug test. He couldn't find anything else wrong, so he assumed I had to be a disgruntled teen who had snuck drugs. Of course, the drug test came back negative, as I never in my life had resorted to taking drugs to cope with my symptoms. Yet again, I was sent home with no answers, left confused and frustrated.

Frustration can be a dangerous place if left there, floundering with no answers.

Uncertainty about your health can also lead to heightened anxiety. Not knowing what's causing the symptoms or how to manage them can create a sense of fear and worry about the future. Many times, in my experience, heightened anxiety accompanying an undiagnosed illness often manifests in additional physical symptoms, intensifying the already overwhelming burden of uncertainty and discomfort.

Physical symptoms would pop up on and off throughout my childhood. Some events were intense, and others were manageable. I do not remember much of my childhood without a migraine present. I also spent a large amount of my time being tested to try to track down answers to the wondering question, what was wrong with me?

I had every test imaginable. I was tested for seizures, heart trouble, vision problems, low blood sugar, cancer... the list goes on. No set of testing came back with answers as to why I had the symptoms. To look at me, I was a happy and healthy young child. Time and again throughout this process, people accused me of making up my symptoms for attention, accused my parents of being paranoid.

When medical professionals cannot offer any reassurances about the cause of your illness, it can trigger a profound sense of loss of control. You find yourself unable to regulate how you feel, and the uncertainty of not having a diagnosis further compounds this feeling of helplessness. Not knowing what's happening to your body can make you feel like you've lost control over your life. This loss of autonomy led me to feelings of powerlessness that were deeply unsettling.

This quickly led to feelings of isolation and guilt for me in my young mind. Living with an undiagnosed illness can be isolating. It is difficult to explain to others what you're going through, and some people do not fully understand or believe your experiences. This isolation can also lead to experiencing guilt. In such moments, it's common to wrestle with guilt and self-blame, questioning why you can't manage daily tasks or meet expectations. The pressure to keep up appearances, to soldier on despite feeling unwell, only adds to the weight of these emotions. It is important, if you find yourself in this position, to reach out to those around you.

Do not let yourself stay trapped in isolation; it can pave the way to a perilous descent into depression.

Living with a chronic illness, particularly when it's undiagnosed, can deeply affect mental well-being. The relentless battle and absence of answers can breed feelings of sadness, hopelessness, and despair. Instead of allowing these dangerous thoughts to enter your mind, replace them with thoughts of hope. While it's important to acknowledge the challenges you face, it's equally crucial to embrace the potential for growth, healing, and the promise of better days ahead. Embracing this perspective can provide strength and motivation to navigate through difficult times with optimism and resilience.

TO MAINTAIN A FEELING OF HOPE, SOMETIMES IT TAKES HAVING A SUPPORT SYSTEM TO FIGHT FOR YOU WHEN YOU CANNOT.

Throughout my young years, my mother stayed fierce. She never stopped attempting to find what appeared to be a nonexistent mystery disease. When the doctors stopped trying to find out what was wrong with me, she proceeded to find new doctors. Due to my mother's persistence, she did find what could have become a life-threatening issue. As an older teenager, I was presenting new symptoms. Where my mother could have ignored them, writing them off as the strange happenings of my childhood, she chose to pursue figuring out what was wrong. Come to find out, I had the presence of a tubular adenoma in my colon, which, for my age, was unheard of. Due to these findings, I was enrolled in some of the first genetics testing out of Washington University in St. Louis, Missouri. Dr. Dayna Early was one of the first doctors to take a firm interest in figuring out what was going on in my young body. She was not willing to take happenstance as an answer. To this day, I still have routine colonoscopies. The first one directly resulted in my still being alive and here today! I also continue to have routine genetic testing to connect more dots as further information becomes available. My hope is to inspire you to find encouragement to never give up the fight to uncover answers. Sometimes, amid a long list of mysteries, lies the solution. Each discovery paves the way to the right diagnosis.

I did not realize it as a child, although looking back, I see now that when dealing with a chronic illness, it is crucial to have someone fighting for you. Someone who believes in you when everyone else writes you off. My illness was not discovered until many years later when I was thirty-five years old, and I was diagnosed with idiopathic intracranial hypertension (IIH), also previously referred to as pseudotumor cerebri. More about that diagnosis later, though. I had many more years ahead of me trying to figure out why sometimes I felt completely normal and other times I barely felt like living.

What part of unraveling the diagnosis are you currently living in? I am deeply grateful to have you alongside me as we navigate the pages of this book together. My sincere wish is that you discover within these words the encouragement and resilience to continue pressing forward in your personal journey. Know that your illness does not define who you are or who you were created to be. With or without the illness, you have a purpose, and you are leaving a footprint on this world in which we live. Each of us carries a narrative worth sharing. Join me as I share my own journey through chronic illness, and may it serve to uplift and empower you wherever you find yourself in your own narrative.

2

BLISSFUL IGNORANCE... OR NOT SO BLISSFUL

"But those who trust in the LORD will find new strength.
They will soar high on wings like eagles. They will run
and not grow weary. They will walk and not faint."

— ISAIAH 40:31 (NLT)

As I started to climb into my early twenties, I stopped chasing the idea that something was wrong and stepped into a season of assuming it was just how I was going to live. Life zoomed forward at lightning-fast speed. I became a young mother and finished my undergrad in finance and financial planning, followed by my master's in business administration and marketing. I tried to push through the bad days as if nothing was wrong. This was no small feat, as at that point, I was living with immense migraines with aura six or seven days a week. These migraines would make me physically sick, lose my vision for small windows of time, were accompanied by intense eye pressure, and would, at times, make me feel as though I was going to pass out.

I determined at that point that I had no choice but to continue forward and proceed as if nothing was wrong. This is no easy task when you feel so extremely ill. However, at that point, I was a young wife and mother to a beautiful young daughter. I did not want my husband to think he had married someone who was broken and unable to function in life, so I hid how badly I felt from him for years. In retrospect, that was a very bad decision. It would have been much better to have been transparent and honest so he could have supported and encouraged me along my journey. As I have learned through the years, having a supportive community while living with a chronic illness is of the utmost importance. We were not created to wade through the sludge of life alone. When we choose to try to do it in our own strength is when we fall into dangerous mental and physical pitfalls.

I WANT TO TAKE A MOMENT TO PAUSE HERE AND SAY, AT THIS POINT IN THE JOURNEY, NOT EVERY DAY WAS MISERABLE.

I even had small windows of time that I felt completely normal. I am now aware that those were times I had gone into remission. I will say, though, before I knew what was going on and about remissions that I had, many times, truly felt I was going insane. As anyone who lives with a chronic illness knows, it is hard not to wonder how it is an illness if it can come and go and change levels of intensity. Our minds are programmed to think if you're sick, you're sick, and if you're well, then you're well, but not a mixture of the two. It has taken years of living with my diagnosis to understand there is a balance between the two when living with a chronic illness.

Learning your body becomes a large piece of that understanding process.

You may discover yourself slipping into the mindset I found myself in during this phase of my journey—brushing aside the evidence that something is wrong and attempting to forge ahead with life. I can share from experience that this is not a healthy mindset for you or anyone around you. When you disregard symptoms, you risk letting underlying health concerns grow and worsen over time. What may seem like a minor issue initially could escalate into something more serious if left unchecked. Many health conditions carry the potential for complications if not addressed promptly. Ignoring symptoms heightens the chances of experiencing these complications, which can prove challenging to manage and treat effectively. This will be what unravels in my personal story as we tread deeper into the mystery of diagnosing my IIH.

Unchecked health issues do not just affect your physical well-being; they also impact your daily life and emotional state.

Symptoms can intensify, leading to discomfort, pain, and limitations in your activities. Neglecting your health can take a toll on your mental and emotional health. The anxiety, stress, and uncertainty stemming from avoiding medical care and confronting potential health issues can weigh heavily on your mind and spirit. I was starting to realize that this was becoming my reality.

Moving further into my journey to find my diagnosis, I had been diagnosed with endometriosis prior to trying for a second child and PCOS later. The doctor had proceeded with doing a laparoscopy to diagnose and treat the endometriosis and better my chances at becoming pregnant. It took several rounds of Lupron shots, post-laparoscopy, to become pregnant with my second daughter. It was a rough pregnancy that resulted in multiple trips to the hospital, thinking the baby was going to come early. I was put on limited activity, which ultimately resulted in a full-term pregnancy. I subsequently delivered the most beautiful and precious baby girl. We were now a family of four, and I could not be more elated! What was even more exciting was after having my second daughter, I went into a small window of remission and was able to enjoy a season that was relatively pain-free and doctor-visit free.

During this time, I had a few life experiences that led me to a different career direction. My goal switched from that of working in business to one focused on helping women escape human sex trafficking. I will have to save that story for another book. My husband and I decided for me to change paths, I needed more education on the topic. So, we moved from our beautiful home in Tupelo, Mississippi, to Lexington, Kentucky, for me to attend Asbury Seminary and later achieve my master's in intercultural studies. It was during this transition that my symptoms began to emerge again. This time they were more intense than before, and I had to seek help for the migraines. When I went to the migraine specialist, they presented me with a few options, one of which included injecting Botox to try to help curb my daily migraines. I did not have an easy feeling about this option. If there is one thing I have learned through this process, it is to lean into God through prayer first and, most importantly, listen to my gut instincts before proceeding. I opted instead of Botox to be put on topiramate. This is a common medication for seizures, nerve pain management, and migraines. What I did not know at the time is this medication is often used in the management of IIH. I found that while being on this medication, my migraines did improve significantly over time, and I felt much relief.

Several years passed, and I would not say I went into remission again, but my symptoms were more managed.

THAT IS, UNTIL 2019, WHEN THE BIGGEST BLESSING AND STORM SEASON I HAD YET FACED BEGAN.

In the summer of 2019, I was told I was pregnant with our third child. This came with so much excitement, as we did not believe we would be able to have another child. Within a month of finding out we were pregnant, we were told the devastating news we had lost the baby. The emotions surrounding this came in waves. We had been told the best and worst news, all within one month's time.

Shortly after, as our emotions were trying to level out, we found out we were yet again pregnant. We proceeded cautiously with this news. We wanted so badly to be elated but were terrified all at the same time. All the "what ifs" were running through our minds.

Then one month, two months, three months passed, and we were still carrying a thriving pregnancy. I had to go off my migraine medication during my pregnancy and soon found myself beginning to plummet physically. I was having more bad days than good days. The pregnancy was really beginning to take a toll on my body.

At sixteen weeks, I started having contractions and was placed on bed rest. I came to find out I had both placenta previa and vasa previa, which is a very rare occurrence. According to the international vasa previa foundation, if it had gone undiagnosed, the fetal mortality rate with this condition is as high as 95 percent.

I was placed on bed rest at home until I reached twenty-nine weeks, then had to continue my bed rest in the hospital. If you're doing the math on the timeline of years here, yes, this was during the initial onset of the COVID-19 pandemic, and due to that, I was not allowed more than one visitor. Thankfully, my husband had come to visit on the exact day our little baby boy decided to make his dramatic entrance into the world. They had me in a hospital room directly beside the delivery room since to save both the baby and me, they would have to deliver the baby at record speed.

I remember vividly what felt like hectic chaos, and I heard things like, "You're losing a lot of blood" and "We have to move now." In the insanity, the doctor on call that night took two seconds to grab my hand and look me in the eye. She said, "I know this is not what you want, but we have to deliver this baby now to keep you and him alive. It is going to be okay." What doctors do not always realize, this one did. Having that small moment calmed my nerves, and off we went.

As they whisked us into the delivery room, the urgency in the air was palpable. I lay there, feeling a mix of fear and anticipation, surrounded by a flurry of activity. The medical team moved swiftly, their voices a blend of reassurance and urgency. In that whirlwind of chaos, I caught a glimpse of my husband's face, his eyes creating a sense of calm amid the storm. His hand on my head was a steady anchor, grounding me in the moment.

"Just breathe," he whispered, his voice a soothing melody in the noise. "It's all going to be okay. We've got this."

As the anesthesiologist administered the medication, a wave of panic washed over me. The sensation of not being able to breathe gripped me, a primal fear seizing my chest. "Am I breathing?" I gasped, my voice trembling with uncertainty. "I don't feel like I can breathe." His response was immediate, his tone unwaveringly calm. "You're breathing," he assured me, his words a lifeline in the darkness of my fear. "You're doing great."

And in that moment, as his words wrapped around me like a warm blanket, I found the strength to believe him. He continued to talk me through every step the doctors were taking, and as I focused on his voice, the panic began to ebb away, replaced by a quiet resolve.

What felt like seconds later, they had successfully delivered my 3.11-pound perfect baby boy. Since the hospital I was in had no room in their NICU, my husband and baby had to be immediately sent to another hospital. Five weeks later, my sweet five-pound baby boy was able to come home and make us a family of five.

In reflection of your own story, either with chronic illness or as a caregiver to someone with a chronic illness, do you find when you look back, it was the wildest roller-coaster ride of your life? Isn't that life, though, enjoying the high points to give you the energy to maintain life during the lows? If there is one thing I have continued to learn in this medical journey of chronic illness, it is to take time to appreciate the positive moments, no matter how small. Gratitude can help shift your focus from challenges to blessings. Maintaining a positive mindset is crucial when dealing with a lifelong struggle.

3

UNDERSTANDING YOUR BODY

*"Come to me, all of you who are weary and carry heavy
burdens, and I will give you rest."*

— MATTHEW 11:28 (NLT)

L iving with a chronic illness necessitates a profound understanding of your own body, a journey that often unfolds as a blend of self-discovery and medical education. In this intricate landscape, awareness transcends mere familiarity with symptoms; it delves into the nuanced rhythms, triggers, and limitations unique to each individual. Navigating daily life becomes an intricate dance, where you learn to decipher the subtle whispers of the body's signals amid the clamor of persistent health challenges. This journey demands patience, resilience, and an unwavering commitment to self-care, as well as an ongoing dialogue between you and your healthcare team. Embracing this journey requires a holistic approach that encompasses physical, emotional, and psychological well-being, ultimately empowering you to reclaim agency over your health while forging a path towards acceptance and adaptation.

It was during this stage of my personal journey that I found my voice as a self-advocate. I initiated the practice of maintaining a symptom journal, recognizing its pivotal role in managing my health. Chronicling symptoms daily, from their intensity and duration to potential triggers, became an indispensable tool. Through this meticulous recordkeeping, patterns gradually surfaced, shedding light on the intricate dynamics of my condition. Vigilance became my ally as I learned to heed the subtle cues my body communicated, whether through pain, fatigue, or shifts in mood. Embracing rest as a form of self-care became crucial, a reminder to honor my body's limits rather than succumb to overexertion.

AT THIS STAGE, I STARTED TO NOTICE NEW SYMPTOMS PAIRED WITH MY DAILY MIGRAINES.

With the uncertainty of COVID-19, I attributed most of my symptoms to either side effects of the vaccine or lingering effects from having had COVID-19. It was not until the summer of 2022 that the symptoms were becoming so unbearable I had to start seeking help. I had developed pulsatile tinnitus in my right ear. It was such a loud sound, like a heartbeat or the ocean. Its intensity had reached a debilitating level, encroaching upon my ability to carry out even the simplest daily tasks. Nights became an endless struggle as the relentless noise deprived me of sleep, offering no respite or escape. I vividly recall moments of desperation, tears streaming down my face as I clutched my ear, yearning for a moment of tranquility. In those agonizing moments, the only solace I craved was the elusive embrace of silence.

One night I remember sitting on the edge of the bed, telling my husband, "I can't take it anymore; it's just too much," my voice choked with emotion.

My husband sat beside me, concern etched on his face as he reached out to comfort me. "I know, sweetheart. It breaks my heart to see you in so much pain." His words were a soothing balm to my wounded soul.

Choking back sobs, I said, "I just want it to stop. I can't remember the last time I had a moment of peace."

His arms wrapped around me, attempting to offer comfort. "I wish I could take the pain away, but please know that I'm here for you, no matter what."

Resting my head on his shoulder, I found a brief respite from the turmoil raging inside me. "I don't know how much longer I can endure this. It feels like I'm drowning in the noise." The weight of my suffering was heavy upon my shoulders that night.

His gentle touch soothed my frayed nerves as he whispered, "We'll figure this out together. We'll find ways to manage it, I promise."

Taking a deep breath, I tried to calm the storm raging within me. "I just need some peace, even if it's just for a moment." I was desperately pleading, seeking refuge in his unwavering presence.

He could sense my desperation, and he pulled me closer, his voice soft and reassuring. "We'll create that moment of peace, whatever it takes. You're not alone in this. I'm right here by your side," he said.

In moments of overwhelming pain and despair, having friends or loved ones by your side can make all the difference. Their unwavering support and empathy serve as pillars of strength when you feel like you're crumbling under the weight of your suffering. Their comforting presence reminds you that you're not alone in your struggles, that there are hands reaching out to lift you up when you can't hold yourself up. They offer a listening ear, a shoulder to lean on, and a heart full of compassion, helping to carry the burden when it becomes too much to bear alone. In their embrace, you find solace, courage, and resilience, knowing that no matter how dark the night may seem, you have allies in the battle against pain and adversity. It's a reminder of the profound importance of human connection, of the healing power of love and empathy in times of greatest need.

Symptoms began progressing at a quicker rate and I experienced such things as head pain, eye pressure, stiffness in my head and neck and down my spine, vision blackouts, eye floaters, optic nerve pressure, loss of balance, dizziness, twitching eyes and other muscles, brain fog including loss of thoughts and words, difficulty speaking at times, disturbance to head and eyes with change in pressure from sneezing or bending over or even going to the bathroom, dehydration, chest pain, joint pain and swelling, nausea, lack of sleep, constant fatigue including extreme heaviness in limbs, bruising, leaking spinal fluid from nose and eyes and ears, loss of motor skills such as dropping what is being held, and others. My life as I once knew it had completely changed at this point, and I was left sitting in a pile of rubble that used to be my life.

HAVE YOU BEEN HERE?

Stunned by the change in your life and not quite sure where to head next. This is the pivotal moment where you can choose one of two diverging paths. Either sit and wallow in your misery or start fighting for your life. Do you ever feel like you do not have it in you to take even one more step? A new doctor, a new diagnosis, new medication to try, all ending in the same results. Do you ever feel defeated and angry, like life has dealt you an unfair hand? Do you ever feel as though all your money is going to medical bills and all your time to appointments, procedures, surgeries, and medications? Do you ever question why and if it is even worth it anymore?

I began asking all these questions and having to force myself to see the why some days. The answer to the questions is simply because it was keeping me alive. It was giving me one more day to be a wife and a mother, a teacher and a friend. It was giving me more time to keep doing what God placed me on this earth to do. I had sunk into a pit of feeling sorry for myself. I had to pull myself together and find my reason for continuing to push forward and fight for answers.

It would just so happen, as I was feeling so overwhelmed with my own symptoms, that would be the time everything around me would soar out of control. It was the start of a new semester in my piano studio, which always comes with extra hours of work and scheduling chaos. My oldest daughter was in her senior year of high school, and application deadlines for college were fast approaching. We had started renovating the upstairs of our home, and our youngest child had a deep eye infection. It is in these moments when you feel the pressure of just one more thing and you are going to crack, throw in the towel, give up.

Isn't that how it all happens, though? Some weeks, we can do nothing more than literally find the strength to take one foot and move it forward. Are you having one of those weeks, maybe even one of those months or years? Don't stop, don't give up. Today is just a small moment in the rest of your life. There is always light at the end of the tunnel. Some tunnels are just a little longer to get through. You do have a purpose; you have a reason to fight. Keep finding the strength to put one foot down in front of you, even if it takes all day to move that one foot.

4

DISCOVERING ANSWERS—WHAT DO YOU DO WITH THEM

"Don't worry about anything; instead, pray about everything. Tell God what you need, and thank him for all he has done. Then you will experience God's peace, which exceeds anything we can understand. His peace will guard your hearts and minds as you live in Christ Jesus."

— PHILIPPIANS 4:6–7 (NLT)

During one of my frequent doctor appointments, the weight of my symptoms seemed to hang heavy in the air. As I sat there, my doctor glanced up from his notes, his expression filled with genuine sympathy. "I truly am sorry," he began, his voice soft with compassion. "You're far too young to be dealing with one of these symptoms, let alone all of them, and for so long." His words resonated deeply within me, a reminder of the unfairness of my circumstances. Can you relate to this? Living with a chronic illness feels as though your entire body is fighting against you. It is like you are living on a daily battlefield striving each day to make it to the next.

I had made an appointment with my family care doctor after spending a large amount of time researching others with similar symptoms. I had found a doctor in New York who did surgeries to place stents and help ease or even stop, in some instances, the sound from the pulsatile tinnitus. I had reached out to the doctor, and he was willing to take me as a patient, but I needed to have some more tests first. He requested I have an MRA and MRV with contrast; then we could discuss further the possibility if I was a candidate for surgery. As I later found out, this specific doctor did not take my insurance, and I was left to find a new doctor to do the same procedure. I was very blessed, after much research, to find a talented neurosurgeon in my own city, Dr. Dashti, who had done research on IIH and had experience with the needed surgery.

While waiting for the tests to be run, I had one of the worst weeks with the pulsatile tinnitus to that point. I sat up in bed in tears and told my husband I was ready to give up. The sound in my head was so loud at this point I could barely function. I was unable to sleep that entire night because of the sound. It was a very long and trying week. The thing with living with a chronic illness is that some days, no matter how hard you try to stay positive, can feel unbearable.

It is in these moments we have to find our reason to fight.

The beauty of continuing to push forward and fight is for the moments of relief that follow the days of despair. The weekend following my very challenging week, I was blessed with seven minutes of silence." At this moment, I was nine months into experiencing the constant symptoms of pulsatile tinnitus. I had not experienced silence in my ear since that specific symptom had begun. I had seven whole minutes pain-free and in complete silence. I was scared to move or even breathe, afraid the moment would go away. I just laid there soaking in the brief reprieve I was being blessed with. It was like God was whispering to me, "Keep going, don't give up." This was the first seven minutes of silence I had heard in nine months and was just the break I needed to continue pushing forward.

The time had come to finally get answers, or so I thought. I went in for the MRA and MRV brain scans and anxiously awaited the results from the radiologist. When I received the call, I quickly scanned over the results overview. Only to read words like normal range, and no issues detected. The feeling of despair quickly swept over my body. I, of course, did not desire something to be wrong with me. The issue was I had the symptoms saying something was wrong, so I desperately desired the answer to what it might be. This made me feel as though I was back, yet again, at square one.

IT WAS AT THIS MOMENT, DUE TO ONE DOCTOR'S CONCERN, I HAD A TURNING POINT.

A moment I will forever be thankful for in my long search for the correct diagnosis. Dr. Stuart Young, an amazing eye doctor in Shelbyville, Kentucky, was having coffee with my husband one morning. As they were finishing their coffee meeting, he asked my husband about what was going on with me. He had read a few posts on Facebook of things I had recently been struggling with. After hearing what all had been happening from my husband, he requested I call and make an appointment with him as soon as possible. He had read some research on an illness that lined up with my symptoms, and he wanted to check my eyes to confirm.

Within that same week, I had my appointment with him. He checked my eyes to find pressure on the optic nerve, confirming his hypothesis. His suggestion was to send me to Bennett and Bloom in Louisville, Kentucky, for a second opinion. Dr. Bloom evaluated my eyes, confirming Dr. Young's possible diagnosis, but needed a spinal tap to fully confirm. Over the course of the following month, additional tests were ordered. I underwent an MRI, CT angiogram, CT temporal bone, spinal tap, and numerous tests on my eyes. All of these tests were sent to my new neurosurgeon, Dr. Dashti, at the Louisville Neuroscience Institute.

There have been specific moments in my care when key doctors have played a crucial role in propelling the advancement of figuring out what I was dealing with physically. I am humbled that Dr. Young took the time to personally take an interest in my case. If it were not for him, my illness might have never been found, and the possibility of me losing my vision from the pressure on my optic nerve would have been great. Doctors with this kind of empathy, commitment to their patients, and concern will always be the reason I continue to push and fight for answers. They give us hope that an answer is out there when all others have given up on us.

Have you been at the point where all hope seems lost, then you receive a little glimmer of hope?

That hope is what you hold on to in the hard times to get you through to the next glimmer. The biggest lesson I have learned from living with a chronic illness is you have to take the mountaintop moments with the valleys. The upcoming months were going to be filled with a little of both as I finally received my diagnosis.

When I went in for the spinal tap, I was full of anticipation and nervousness, as I knew this was going to be one of the bigger factors in a diagnosis. Upon completion of the procedure, the doctor proceeded to tell me the pressure going into my brain was at 40 cm h2o and the normal range was 6-15 cm h2o. It was the highest level of pressure he had personally seen in conducting spinal taps. He went on to tell me he had drained the spinal fluid from 40 down to 15, which should provide relief for a short time until the spinal fluid began rising again in my head. I immediately felt relief. I felt like a new person. I wanted to jump off that hospital bed and start running a marathon. However, if you have had a spinal tap, you know that is not advised. So, as good as I felt, I had to stay lying flat on my back until completely healed from the procedure to not cause complications.

As we left the hospital, I was so elated by the relief I was feeling. I was not hearing the ocean sound in my ear; I had no pain or pressure pushing on my eyes. My headache was gone, and my mind felt clear. Sadly, the relief I felt lasted no longer than three hours, and all my symptoms came back like a flood. The devastation I felt as the symptoms hit is almost indescribable. I experienced life nearly pain-free and had a small glimpse of what I could possibly feel like, only to have it taken away as quickly as it came.

IN THE AFTERMATH, MY MIND SWIRLED WITH CONFLICTING EMOTIONS.

Hope, so briefly ignited, now flickered dimly in the recesses of my consciousness, overshadowed by the overwhelming despair of my symptoms returning. Questions danced inside my thoughts, taunting me with their unanswerable nature. Why couldn't the relief last? Would I ever experience true respite from this relentless torment? The brief taste of normalcy only served to deepen the ache of longing within me, a yearning for a life unencumbered by the shackles of chronic illness. And yet, amid the darkness of my despair, a spark of determination flickered defiantly. I had felt the fleeting touch of relief, however brief, and it was enough to fuel my resolve to keep fighting, to cling to the hope that one day, I might find a lasting reprieve from the prison of my own body.

Due to the fast recurrence of symptoms, I was placed on Diamox immediately and diagnosed with progressive idiopathic intracranial hypertension (IIH), also known as pseudotumor cerebri. The medication was an attempt to save my vision and hopefully relieve some pressure from my brain where the spinal fluid was essentially keeping my brain in a vise. Sadly, the medication came with its own side effects I was not prepared for. One specific side effect I found fascinating. I remember asking my doctor if the medicine would alleviate the ocean sound in my ear, during which he told me if they leveled it out to the right dosage, the sound should stop. After the first day of medication, I discovered not an ocean sound, but a loud ringing in not one but both my ears. I reached out to the doctor about this new symptom and his response, I have to admit, made me chuckle out loud. He said, "Oh, ringing in the ears can be a side effect of this medication." This had to be the epitome of my journey with chronic illness so far. Sometimes you just have to take a moment and laugh so you do not cry. It would appear I had traded an ocean sound for ringing, which seemed like a linear transition in my opinion, but a step forward in progress, at least according to the medical community.

Do you remember a time in the process of your diagnosis when you felt excitement and exhaustion all in the same breath? This was one of those times for me in my journey. It was fantastic I finally had a diagnosis, but still overwhelming to have no answers as to the cause or a cure.

5

A DAY IN THE LIFE WITH HANK

"Each time he said, "My grace is all you need. My power works best in weakness." So now I am glad to boast about my weaknesses, so that the power of Christ can work through me."

— 2 CORINTHIANS 12:9 (NLT)

Hank, the mischievous troublemaker, made his grand entrance into our lives courtesy of my imaginative children. Picture this: We're cruising down the road on our usual weekly drive when, lo and behold, I miss our exit. "Where are we going, Mom?" pipes up my youngest daughter, genuinely puzzled.

"To dance class, sweetheart," I reply, completely oblivious to my blunder.

"Um, Mom, you just missed the exit," my eldest points out, trying to stifle a giggle. And then, without skipping a beat, she declares, "Oh, Mom, it's Hank messing with your head again, isn't it?"

Confused, I ask, "Who in the world is Hank?"

Cue uproarious laughter from both kids as they explain that Hank is the imaginary troublemaker they've named for the havoc my IIH brings. And just like that, Hank becomes the scapegoat for every silly symptom-induced mishap in our lives, adding a touch of whimsy to our everyday adventures.

SO LET ME TAKE YOU ON A JOURNEY AS A TYPICAL DAY IN THE LIFE WITH HANK.

As the sun timidly peeks through the curtains, signaling the dawn of a new day, I open my eyes to greet the world. But before I can fully embrace the day, I am met with the familiar presence of Hank, as my children so lovingly named him.

He is my constant companion and formidable adversary— my IIH-induced brain fog, memory eraser, and vision stealer.

The morning begins with a delicate dance of determination and resilience. It begins with the simple struggle to crawl out of bed. What seems like an ordinary task for most is quite possibly the hardest for those of us living with IIH. As I move to sit up, the pressure increases in my head, causing a flood of pain to my body. The pulsatile tinnitus in my ear begins yelling loudly, my head throbs like it might explode off my shoulders, and when I open my eyes, I stare through what appears to be polka dots and party confetti sprinkled in my vision as eye floaters taint my view. Simple tasks like getting out of bed and preparing breakfast are shrouded in a thick fog, as if the world itself is obscured by a veil of uncertainty. Yet, with each step forward, I refuse to succumb to the challenges that Hank presents.

Navigating through the day is a changing adventure, with Hank as the elusive lurking monster around every corner. Concentration becomes a fleeting luxury, as thoughts scatter like leaves in the wind, making it difficult to grasp on to even the simplest of ideas. Yet, I persist, armed with patience and an unwavering resolve to reclaim control over my mind, along with pushing through the pain that seems to attack my body constantly.

Walking appears to be one of the larger struggles. My feet stay in a constant state of being swollen and bruised, making it difficult to place pressure on them. My joints hurt, and my body is heavy, as if I have just completed running the biggest marathon of my life. Upon making my coffee, I hobble into the living room to sit and raise my feet to relieve some of the morning pain before launching into my brisk morning of preparing my children's breakfast and starting their studies for the day. At this point, I have been out of bed less than an hour, and already my body needs a break. Imagine with me a moment, being a young and vibrant woman with so much life still ahead of you and having to take a break because your body said getting out of bed was simply too much for the day.

Every interaction becomes a delicate balancing act as I grapple with the unpredictable nature of my condition.

Conversations stutter and stall, as words slip through my grasp like grains of sand. Yet, amid the frustration and confusion, there are moments of clarity—brief glimpses of the person I once was shining through the fog like beacons of hope. Despite the challenges that Hank presents, I refuse to let IIH define me. With each passing hour, I find solace in the small victories—the moments of clarity, the flickers of inspiration—that remind me of the strength that lies within.

As I progress through my day, my body starts to tighten. The back of my head feels swollen and painful, like two knots have formed at the base of my head. My shoulders and down over my spine fill with pain when I sit or move. The ocean sound in my ear whooshes louder and louder with every movement, causing more confusion in my thoughts as I strive to focus past the noise. I pause to place my hands over my eyes. The pain behind my eyes is not describable. At best, it feels as though something is trying to push on my eyes from the inside. They call it an optic migraine, although it feels as though Hank has come at my eyes with a vengeance. I blink and blink again. My vision goes black. Just for a short moment, but it was definitely gone. When it returns, my vision is filled with floaters, yet another symptom that makes it a struggle to maintain my sanity during the day.

The requirements of me within my day are starting to weigh heavy within the battle my body is fighting. I am still a wife and a mother with responsibilities like cooking, cleaning, homeschooling, and, more importantly, just being present in my family's lives. I own my own business in which I am responsible for close to one hundred students to properly train them in piano education. I have friends and family who depend on me to join them in daily life. I play piano for our church. I assist in nonprofit work as needed. I attempt to be there for others and their battles as often as I can, knowing how healing it is to be there for people.

I do my best to hide and conceal the inner battle raging in my life, so others are not affected negatively by the daily struggles I face.

Meanwhile, as my day progresses, it is now time to begin teaching. I feel the telltale signs of my condition escalating. With a subtle yet persistent pressure building in my head, I find myself instinctively reaching to wipe away the moisture from my eyes, nose, and ears. It's a ritual I've become all too familiar with—a signal that I've reached a critical juncture in my day. The relentless accumulation of spinal fluid within my skull has reached a tipping point, seeking its own avenue of escape. As I strive to maintain focus on the task at hand, I'm acutely aware of the mounting pressure within, threatening to overwhelm my senses and disrupt the delicate balance of my teaching routine. Despite the discomfort and distraction, I soldier on, determined to fulfill my responsibilities and provide my students with the education they deserve. Yet, with each passing moment, the physical manifestations of my condition serve as a stark reminder of the challenges I face daily.

At this moment, I am filled with gratitude for the small, cherished circle of individuals with whom I can be entirely authentic and vulnerable. They are my refuge on the most challenging of days— those who extend a caring hand to inquire about my well-being, both physically and emotionally. They are the ones who offer prayers, lending their strength to mine, and who leave gentle reminders of their love and support, such as flowers at my doorstep, brightening even the darkest of moments. They are the ones who ease the burdens of daily life by preparing a meal and lifting the weight from my weary shoulders. Without the unwavering support and encouragement of my inner circle, this journey would feel nearly insurmountable.

As the day draws to a close and the world is bathed in the gentle glow of twilight, I reflect on the journey I have undertaken. Hank may be a formidable adversary, but he is also a testament to my strength—a constant reminder of the power within me to endure, even in the face of adversity. As I prepare to face another day with Hank by my side, I do so with a newfound sense of purpose and determination, ready to confront whatever challenges lie ahead. For in the battle against IIH, every day is a victory—a testament to the courageous spirit that resides within us all.

QUESTIONS FOR REFLECTION

Do you find yourself currently in a situation that feels unbearable? What is it? Give words to what is making you feel as though your life has been reduced to nothing more than rubble.

Now take a moment to write down everything that feels hopeless. Is it physical, mental, emotional, financial, or spiritual stress weighing you down? Try to use one-word descriptions here.

Of your list above, what is one thing you can let go of? This is not an easy step. Sometimes, we see our list and see no way out. You obviously cannot let go of a physical ailment, but you can let go of how it is controlling your constant thoughts.

For example: I am choosing today to let go of my constant focus on the ocean sound in my ear and instead replace my thoughts with positives I definitely have in my life. I am thankful this day to have a roof over my head, or I am thankful for a specific friend or family member. Be as specific as you can in your gratitude.

PART TWO
MANAGING SYMPTOMS: DOCTORS, TREATMENTS, SURGERIES, STRATEGIES

6

NAVIGATING MEDICAL CARE: EMPOWERING YOURSELF THROUGH KNOWLEDGE

"Don't be afraid, for I am with you. Don't be discouraged, for I am your God. I will strengthen you and help you. I will hold you up with my victorious right hand."

— ISAIAH 41:10 (NLT)

I f I hear one more person say, "Just lose weight, and you will feel better," I might scream. If I had a dollar for every time I have been told this condition primarily affects overweight females, so just lose weight, and you will feel better, then I would be a millionaire. In the complex world of idiopathic intracranial hypertension, understanding the complexities of this condition is important to navigating its challenges effectively. Characterized by elevated pressure within the skull without an identifiable cause, IIH presents a unique set of hurdles for patients and healthcare providers alike. In this journey through the corridors of medical care, empowerment through knowledge becomes not just a tool, but a lifeline. From deciphering treatment options to advocating for personalized care, the ability to navigate the healthcare system and arm oneself with understanding is instrumental. My hope is that this section serves as a guide traversing the often-daunting landscape of IIH, illuminating the path toward informed decision-making, proactive engagement, and ultimately, improved outcomes. Knowledge is not just power, but the key to reclaiming control in the face of uncertainty.

Due to the nature of the complexities of IIH, the care plan for each person is going to be individualized, making creating a treatment plan even more complex. I have found some steps to be very helpful as I have navigated the road to find one. The first step is to educate yourself as much as you can. This can be done through joining support groups and leaning on help from others who have already walked this road. I am very thankful for the support groups I have found as they have been a huge aid and encouragement, as well as a great resource of information.

DO YOUR RESEARCH

It is important when you are doing your research to make sure to research reputable sources. As we all know, falling into the rabbit hole of online medical research can be more damaging than it is helpful. Take the time to research your condition, treatment options, and any medications prescribed to you. Use reputable sources such as medical journals, trusted websites, or books written by healthcare professionals. This step is a little more challenging when researching IIH as it has limited resources available.

ASK GOOD QUESTIONS

This leads to the importance of the next step, making sure to ask good questions to your medical team. Don't hesitate to ask your healthcare provider questions about your condition, treatment plan, or any concerns you may have. Write down your questions beforehand to ensure you don't forget anything during your appointment. Thinking through your questions in advance is crucial. With IIH, brain fog is a real challenge, and time with medical staff can be limited, so you want to take full advantage of that time you have.

Structuring your questions for your doctor is important. Begin by introducing yourself and providing context for the appointment, summarizing your medical history related to your current symptoms or concerns. Then, delve into the specifics of your symptoms and inquire about your diagnosis and treatment plan. Seek clarity on medications, potential side effects, and long-term management strategies. This is where not skipping the first part of this process becomes important. You want to go into this appointment with information in hand from your personal research so you can ask the appropriate questions. Discuss the prognosis for your condition and establish a plan for follow-up and monitoring. Allow space for any additional questions or concerns you may have, ensuring that all issues are addressed. By organizing your questions in this structured manner, you can make the most of your time with your doctor and ensure that your healthcare needs are met comprehensively.

GET A SECOND OPINION

In attempting to acquire a correct diagnosis, there are a few other important steps. Many people with IIH are either misdiagnosed or ignored, creating the importance of getting a second opinion. You must remember that you are your biggest advocate. If something is wrong, then you don't stop pushing for answers until you find them. Even if the first doctor gave you a diagnosis, another benefit to getting a second opinion is different perspectives can provide valuable insights and help you make informed decisions about your care.

ADVOCATE FOR YOURSELF

Take an active role in your healthcare by advocating for yourself when necessary. Don't be afraid to speak up if you feel that something isn't right or if you have questions or concerns about your care. You know yourself better than anyone else, which includes knowing when something is amiss. It is important for you to trust your instincts. If something doesn't feel right or if you're not satisfied with your current care, don't hesitate to seek alternative options or advocate for changes. Your intuition and well-being are important factors in navigating medical care effectively.

UNDERSTAND YOUR HEALTH INSURANCE

It is also important if you have health insurance coverage that you take some time to understand what your insurance provider covers. The last thing you want is to find the right doctor or the right procedure and your insurance does not cover you. Familiarize yourself with your health insurance plan, including coverage, co-pays, deductibles, and any preauthorization requirements. This can help you avoid unexpected costs and navigate the financial aspects of medical care more effectively. The road to finding a diagnosis has been paved with countless medical bills year after year. Understanding the cost expectation up front can help in the process of creating a medical plan.

STAY ORGANIZED

My final suggestion is to stay organized. The road to a diagnosis is not a short one for most people. Keep track of appointments, medications, and important documents related to your healthcare in a centralized location. Consider using digital tools or apps to help you stay organized and manage your health information more efficiently. Within only a few months, I had scans from two different doctors on my eyes, a spinal tap, multiple appointments with my general practitioner, two sets of bloodwork, and five different brain scans at three different locations. Without good recordkeeping, it would have been very challenging to collect the appropriate information when the time came for my appointment with my neurosurgeon.

Navigating medical care is a journey entwined with challenges, uncertainties, and complexities. Yet, armed with knowledge, empowerment, and a proactive approach, you can go to battle for yourself with confidence. By educating yourself about your condition, advocating for your needs, and actively participating in your healthcare decisions, you can reclaim a sense of control in your healthcare journey. Moreover, effective communication with healthcare providers, strategic use of resources, and a willingness to seek support and second opinions can further help the navigation process. Ultimately, navigating medical care is not just about reaching a destination; it's about empowering yourself to make informed decisions, advocate for personalized care, and achieve optimal health outcomes. As we continue on this journey, let us remember that knowledge, empowerment, and resilience are our greatest allies in the pursuit of health and well-being.

7

EXAMINING THE OPTIONS

*"Trust in the LORD with all your heart; do not depend on your
own understanding. Seek his will in all you do, and he will
show you which path to take."*

— PROVERBS 3:5–6 (NLT)

The world of IIH comes with an overwhelming
consideration of options, ranging from medicine that
doesn't feel as though it is effective to surgeries that can
sometimes have scary outcomes. Imagine, if you will, the pain in
your head being unbearable, the relentless throbbing punctuating
each moment of your existence. Visual disturbances become your
constant companions, obscuring the world in a haze of blurriness
and shadows. The weight of fatigue settles upon your shoulders,
dragging you into a perpetual state of exhaustion. As much as this
might be the story of one person suffering from the condition, the
next person might have a completely different experience.

However, amid the darkness of uncertainty, glimmers of hope
emerge in the form of treatment options. From medications to
dietary adjustments and surgeries, a myriad of paths stretch before

those seeking relief from the relentless grip of IIH. Each avenue holds its own promises and pitfalls, weaving a complex tapestry of choices for patients and their caregivers to navigate. In this journey through the landscape of IIH treatment, let's explore these options, shedding light on their efficacy, risks, and considerations. Our quest is not merely to enumerate the possibilities, but to empower those of us affected by IIH with knowledge, along with providing the tools necessary to make informed decisions.

I WANT TO TALK ABOUT A FEW OF THE MOST COMMONLY SUGGESTED MEDICATIONS.

This is by no means medical advice; this is just my personal path and the options I chose to try in my journey of IIH. The first medication I was placed on before I had a diagnosis was topiramate, also known as Topamax. I was given this medication for the migraines that were running my life at the time. I had not been given an IIH diagnosis yet. Therefore, my doctors were unaware of what they were treating. It just so happened that the medication they prescribed me, I later found out, was a commonly used medication for IIH migraines. After being on this medication for a few weeks, I began feeling relief from my almost daily migraines. There were some side effects that were challenging, though, including dizziness, sleepiness, nausea, tingling in my arms and legs, and difficulty sleeping. Overall, I found the benefits of this medication outweighed the side effects, as I was able to function more effectively without the disturbance of an intense migraine. This did not do away with my migraines completely, but I was able to go from sometimes six to seven days a week down to one to two days a week of migraines.

Another common medication prescribed for IIH is acetazolamide or Diamox. Doctors tend to prescribe this because it is a diuretic that supposedly reduces cerebrospinal fluid (CSF) production, helping to lower intracranial pressure. One of the biggest reasons to lower the pressure is to save your vision. Pressure on the optic nerve can lead to blindness.

Although there seem to be mixed reviews on this medication from those of us placed on it as a treatment for our condition. Some say it was the catalyst to control the symptoms while others say that it created more symptoms, making living with the condition unbearable. While on Diamox, I experienced a range of side effects that affected my daily life. The medication caused frequent urination, leaving me feeling constantly thirsty and disrupting my sleep with trips to the bathroom throughout the night. I also experienced tingling sensations in my hands and feet, as well as a metallic taste in my mouth, which made eating less enjoyable. Although I had been warned that the carbonation from soda created a nasty metal taste, I suppose I just had to find out for myself. My husband and I had gone out to eat for a date night, and I ordered a root beer with my meal. When I went to take the first drink it came back out about as quickly as it went in. Least to say, they were very accurate in the description of how nasty the medicine made sodas taste. Nausea and occasional vomiting also made it difficult to maintain a regular appetite, contributing to feelings of fatigue and weakness. I often also felt lightheaded and dizzy, especially when standing up quickly, and my vision occasionally became blurred.

Despite these challenges, I found some relief from my symptoms, but the side effects of Diamox made the treatment process a difficult balancing act between managing my condition and coping with its effects on my body. I was not on Diamox long term as it was an interim treatment before surgery, so I did not get to the point of experiencing the medication leveling out in my system. Others have said that over time the symptoms do adjust slightly, making them more bearable.

IMPLEMENTING DIETARY CHANGES AS PART OF MANAGING MY CONDITION INVOLVED A SIGNIFICANT ADJUSTMENT TO MY EATING HABITS.

One of the key changes was restricting my sodium intake, which meant carefully monitoring the salt content of my meals and avoiding high-sodium foods. This adjustment was challenging, as many processed and convenience foods are high in sodium. Doctors also suggested that limiting foods high in vitamin A is important as well.

Additionally, I had to limit my fluid intake, particularly caffeinated and sugary beverages, to help reduce fluid retention and possibly give some relief to symptoms. Incorporating more fruits, vegetables, and whole grains into my diet became essential for maintaining overall health while managing my condition. Despite the initial difficulty in adapting to these dietary changes, I found that they played a crucial role in managing my symptoms and improving my quality of life. Although much of the medical community will insist the best cure for symptoms is simply weight loss, it does seem to be much more complex than that for those of us living with the condition. As many in my support group have lost an extraordinary amount of weight, only to be left with more intense symptoms.

This should not discourage us from having the desire to become a healthy weight, though. Losing weight can bring about a multitude of benefits, both physically and emotionally. Shedding excess pounds can significantly reduce the risk of developing various health conditions such as heart disease, type 2 diabetes, and hypertension. Moreover, weight loss often leads to improved mobility and joint health, relieving strain on the body and enhancing overall physical function. Beyond the physical realm, achieving a healthier weight can boost self-confidence, increase energy levels, and foster a more positive body image, ultimately enhancing our quality of life.

As great as all this sounds, it is much easier said than done.

As someone who spent the largest majority of my life underweight, now having changed the role into experiencing life slightly overweight has been a challenge to adapt to. I have found that weight loss with this condition is simply frustrating at best. I lose one pound to gain back five the following day. It is an uphill struggle to shed any weight, even in the best conditions. I am limited in the activities I do that would lead to weight loss. Anything that would increase pressure in my head only compounds my symptoms, and the risks outweigh the benefits.

It is very challenging to exercise when my body struggles most days to move. Every person with this condition is different, but I have found that less vigorous activity is the best. Committing to daily movement is a good place to start. I walk twenty minutes a day, no matter how I am feeling. Some days that twenty minutes feels like four hours, and other days, it is so enjoyable that I can continue for more time. Swimming is also an excellent option. I have found the water takes the pressure off my body and improves the quality of how I feel. Finding a way to move every day with low impact is such a great start to improving weight control, paired with creating healthy eating habits.

It is also important to address surgical intervention as an option for IIH. Optic nerve sheath fenestration (ONSF) becomes a focal point, symbolizing both the desperation and determination to preserve vision and alleviate debilitating pressure on the optic nerve. However, the journey doesn't end with ONSF; rather, it serves as a catalyst for further exploration of surgical avenues. Ventriculoperitoneal (VP) shunting emerges as a lifeline for those facing the most severe levels of IIH, offering a chance to divert excess cerebrospinal fluid away from the brain and toward the abdomen, where it can be safely absorbed.

Another option for surgery is venous sinus stenting, a cutting-edge procedure offering renewed hope for those with IIH and venous sinus stenosis. Venous sinus stenting is a minimally invasive surgical procedure used to treat conditions affecting the veins within the brain, particularly when there is venous sinus stenosis (narrowing) or thrombosis (blood clotting) that leads to elevated intracranial pressure. This procedure involves placing a small mesh tube, known as a stent, into the affected venous sinus to widen the narrowed area and improve blood flow.

The journey through the landscape of treatments, dietary changes, and surgeries is one filled with challenges, yet brimming with hope. It is a delicate balance of medication regimens, dietary adjustments, and the transformative potential of surgical interventions, each avenue offering a ray of light amid the shadows of uncertainty. In the end, it is through empathy, understanding, and a steadfast commitment to exploring every option that we forge a path toward hope, healing, and the promise of a brighter tomorrow.

8

INTO THE OPERATING ROOM

"Give all your worries and cares to God, for he cares about you."

— 1 PETER 5:7 (NLT)

Emotions, uncertainty, relief, and hope were all running through my mind as I entered Norton Neuroscience to see Dr. Dashti. The decision to undergo surgery was a profound turning point. My path with IIH has been a winding one, marked by the relentless ebb and flow of symptoms and the tireless pursuit of effective treatments. Through the lens of my own experience with venous stenosis coiling, and sharing intimate details of my journey, I hope to provide insight and hope for you if you're considering the same procedure. This narrative is not just a recounting of my personal story; it's a testament to resilience in the face of adversity. As our support group says often, we are strong because we are IIH warriors.

The moment the surgeon mentioned coiling surgery, it felt like a seismic shift in my journey. He spoke with confidence, laying out statistics like breadcrumbs on a path to potential relief. "Eighty percent chance of success," he declared, his voice brimming with assurance. Yet, beneath his confidence lurked the shadows of my own uncertainty—the risks cast a long shadow over his words. Brain bleeds, stroke, sudden death—words that hung heavy in the air, a reminder of the high stakes of this surgical gamble, even if there was low risk. Despite his demeanor, I couldn't shake the gravity of his warnings. "No casualties," he proclaimed, his tone filled with confidence. And perhaps rightly so, for he is a titan in his field, unmatched in his experience with these surgeries across the United States.

Even as he outlined the procedure's efficiency, a chill ran down my spine at the thought of the pain that awaited me.

And if, by some cruel twist of fate, the surgery failed to deliver the promised reprieve, the alternatives loomed before me like ominous shadows. Brain shunts and the relentless dependency on Diamox—a bitter pill to swallow, both figuratively and literally. The surgeon's disdain for these alternatives was palpable, his warning against Diamox ringing in my ears. Yet, in the face of potential blindness, it seemed I had little choice. In the intricate dance of decision-making, uncertainty hung heavy, obscuring the path ahead. But as I stood at the precipice of choice, I knew that whatever lay beyond, my journey with IIH would be forever altered by the weight of this decision.

Have you been in a similar position? The daily struggle of living with the symptoms leads to the weight of considering surgical options. It is like a fine balancing act weighing the potential benefits of the surgery against the potential risks.

With just twenty-four hours until my surgery, my mind was a whirlwind of questions and uncertainties. How would the surgery unfold? Would it bring the relief I've been longing for, or would complications arise? The thought of potential side effects loomed large—would I be forced back onto Diamox, despite its harsh toll on my body? Only two weeks on the medication, and already, signs of severe dehydration and kidney strain were surfacing. Worse yet, it didn't even seem to keep my symptoms at bay effectively.

IN THAT MOMENT, I REALIZED THE POWER OF SHIFTING MY MINDSET.

Dwelling on the uncertainties and potential pitfalls would only serve to erode my confidence and resilience. This is where the true potential of our thoughts comes into play. If we allow ourselves to be consumed by negativity, our entire demeanor will suffer, casting a shadow over our outlook and, potentially, our outcomes.

Maintaining a positive mindset before surgery is pivotal for several reasons. Firstly, it can alleviate anxiety and fear, helping to keep stress levels in check. By focusing on the possibilities of a successful outcome, we can cultivate a sense of calm and inner peace, essential for facing the challenges ahead with clarity and determination.

A positive mindset can bolster our ability to bounce back and ability to cope with setbacks.

Surgery, like any medical procedure, comes with its own set of risks and uncertainties. However, by approaching it with a positive attitude, we can better navigate any obstacles that may arise, maintaining our resolve and determination to persevere.

I found that cultivating a positive mindset had tangible benefits on my physical well-being. Research has shown that optimism and positive thinking can boost the immune system, promote faster recovery, and even reduce the perception of pain. By harnessing the power of positivity, we can optimize our body's ability to heal and recuperate post-surgery.

It is crucial to maintain a positive mindset to foster a sense of empowerment and agency over our circumstances. Instead of feeling powerless in the face of adversity, we can take proactive steps to prepare ourselves mentally and emotionally for the journey ahead. By choosing to focus on hope, gratitude, and resilience, we can approach surgery with a sense of confidence and determination, knowing that we have the strength and resilience to overcome whatever challenges may arise.

The morning of the surgery, I felt such a sense of peace. I had come to terms with my choice to have coiling surgery, and I knew I was in more than capable hands with my surgical team. Before my surgery, I was decked out in the latest fashion: a hospital gown with built-in heating! It was like being wrapped in a toasty burrito of warmth. The only downside? I couldn't take this snazzy warming contraption home with me! Talk about a missed opportunity to be the envy of all my family during movie nights.

Upon completion of the surgery, I opened my eyes, slightly confused about my surroundings as a nurse was standing over me, applying immense pressure to the entry point for my coiling. Waking up to this was not pleasant, and it was very painful. This process had to be repeated two other times in the ICU recovery room as the femoral artery continued to have difficulty clotting.

The haze of pain began to lift, and as I was wheeled into my ICU room, a newfound clarity washed over me. With each passing moment, my senses sharpened, and I found myself focusing on my symptoms. To my amazement, the incessant drumming of pulsatile tinnitus had vanished, leaving behind a blissful silence that soothed my troubled mind. Yet, amid the waves of relief, a different sensation emerged—the most intense head pain I had ever experienced gripped me with merciless force. And yet, there was a strange sense of reassurance. For, despite the pain, I knew that the surgery had achieved its intended success, offering a glimmer of hope amid the storm.

When the doctor made his rounds, he began to go into detail about my procedure, and the gravity of the issue became evident. There was a noticeable drop in pressure in the veins around my brain, specifically an 11 mm Hg decrease at a key junction. Imagine a tube that starts off wide but narrows significantly. This makes it difficult for water to flow through. In my case, the cerebrospinal fluid had trouble moving because the tube was partially blocked. Once a stent was placed, it opened up the blocked area and helped relieve the symptoms. Reflecting on my journey to this point, I realize how crucial it is to confront uncertainty with courage and a positive mindset. The decision to undergo coiling surgery was daunting, filled with the weight of potential risks and the strain of living with IIH. Yet, by focusing on the possibility of relief, I found a strength I didn't know I had.

9

ROAD TO RECOVERY

"He gives power to the weak and strength to the powerless."

— ISAIAH 40:29 (NLT)

As I lay in my hospital bed in the ICU post-surgery, the nurse noticed I had a peaceful smile on my face. She looked at me at one point and asked, "You're one of those who smiles through pain, aren't you?" This was the truest of all statements, but that wasn't why I was smiling at this exact moment. Although I knew the stenting was not a cure for my condition, I did know it brought much relief to some of the most severe of symptoms. For this, I was immensely grateful!

I cannot recount to you the amount of food I consumed post-surgery. I do believe I was the levity of the entire nursing staff on my ICU floor. For those who have experienced the dread of taking Diamox, you know the evil of horrendous taste alteration. The metallic undertones that tainted every drink previously were now gone. In their place emerged a vibrant palette of flavors, a kaleidoscope of delights, and oh, did I enjoy those first few days.

We all take the simplest of things for granted until we no longer have them to enjoy. I was able to taste what I was eating and drinking, in addition to not becoming violently ill every time I put a bite of food in my mouth. Amid the simple joy of eating again, there lingered a profound gratitude—a gratitude for the simple pleasure of flavor.

As I lay in the ICU after my brain-stenting procedure, the night stretched on endlessly, devoid of sleep. The night nurse, a comforting presence in the dimly lit room, made her rounds, her footsteps a steady rhythm in the quiet of the night. "You doing okay?" she asked softly, her voice laced with concern as she checked my memory every hour. "Not much sleep, huh?"

I chuckled weakly, the pain in my head still intense. "Not really," I admitted, trying to find humor in the situation. At one point, she dropped her clipboard, a small moment of clumsiness in the otherwise calm night. "Oh, don't worry," I reassured her with a smile. "You won't wake my husband up. Nothing wakes him."

She laughed softly, glancing over at my peacefully sleeping husband. "I see that. He didn't even budge." Curiosity sparked in her eyes as she observed my upbeat demeanor amid the post-surgery recovery.

"Are you always this positive and happy?" Admiration was evident in her voice.

I shrugged slightly, a faint smile gracing my lips. "I try to be. It helps to focus on the good, especially in times like these."

Throughout the night, we exchanged conversation, the nurse diligently checking on me while I struggled to find respite from the pain and discomfort. As the night wore on and sleep remained elusive, I turned to my praise and worship music, the familiar melodies offering solace and distraction from my restless thoughts. In the quiet of the ICU, amid the beeping machines and hushed whispers,

I found a semblance of peace, my faith guiding me through the darkness of the night.

MORNING TWO GREETED ME WITH A SENSE OF REFRESHED VITALITY, A RARITY IN RECENT MEMORY.

Despite lingering discomfort—a headache persisting, a reminder of the metal now nestled within my brain—I found solace in the promise of healing. Physical fatigue weighed heavily, exacerbated by the sharp pain that still flared with each cough or simple movement, a relentless reminder of the recent surgical intervention. And amid the chaos of sound, my senses remained overwhelmed, struggling to find equilibrium in the wake of the procedure.

Yet, in the middle of these trials, glimmers of hope emerged, casting light on the path ahead.

The incessant pulsatile tinnitus, a constant companion for far too long, had vanished into the quietude of memory. My once-clouded mind, the product of my companion Hank, shrouded in a haze of confusion, now found clarity; I could articulate thoughts with newfound ease, navigating conversations with a renewed sense of focus.

Though pressure lingered behind my eyes, a testament to ongoing healing, the veil of blurry vision had lifted, revealing a world restored to sharp clarity. In the eyes of my loved ones, I glimpsed the subtle shifts brought by the surgeon's skilled hands—an improvement in communication, a return to the fluidity of speech that had eluded me in recent times.

The revelation of a small aneurysm, discovered amid the tangle of vessels, cast a shadow of uncertainty, tempered only by the reassurance of future monitoring. As I navigated the limitations imposed by the healing process—days devoid of driving, lifting, or bending—a sense of purpose guided my actions, a commitment to safeguarding against the potential of further complications.

In the days following my hospital stay, I proceeded to recover from the comfort of my home. Pain management became my biggest focus for the first several days. Navigating balance to prevent extreme fatigue and controlling the noise to prevent noise agitation were of high priority. Recovery was much like life; there were days I felt more like I was on a mountaintop, and others I felt like I was in a valley struggling to climb and make it through the day.

I FOUND MYSELF NAVIGATING UNCHARTED TERRITORY, FILLED WITH BOTH CHALLENGES AND TRIUMPHS.

Each day brought its own set of hurdles, but I was determined to persevere, drawing strength from the support of my loved ones and the stories of strength shared by others who had walked a similar path. My support group continued to be an important part of my recovery process as I leaned on others who had walked this path before me.

As the days progressed, it appeared that my surgery had been a success. For this, I felt an overwhelming sense of gratitude. Days after the surgery, the surgeon reached out to deliver an update and check on my progress, emphasizing the need for ongoing monitoring. While the surgery typically offers a swift resolution, its effectiveness can vary greatly from person to person. Some individuals may find themselves returning for follow-up procedures within as little as four months, while others may progress to the necessity of shunt drains to alleviate pressure from their brains.

Through this process, some realities hung heavy in my mind like a haunting refrain. Thoughts about how I could die or have a stroke or a heart attack, the surgery could fail, or simply be temporary. In the end, the surgery was more of a bandage than a cure. I still had a rare brain condition, for which there is not yet a cure. The gravity of this realization slowly settled in, reminding me of the fragile balance of life.

Was Hank totally gone forever or was he just downgraded from driver to passenger?

IN THE AFTERMATH OF MY SURGERY, ONE MONTH LATER, I FOUND MYSELF CONFRONTING A NEW SET OF CHALLENGES.

My surgeon delivered the sobering news that the symptoms lingering post-operation were likely here to stay. The persistent ringing in both ears, sporadic pressure behind my eyes, and the sensation of plugged ears similar to that of being on a perpetual plane ride became unwelcome companions in my daily life.

Yet, during the frustration and discomfort these symptoms brought, I found solace in the remarkable improvements elsewhere. The absence of pulsatile tinnitus in my right ear was a small victory amid the larger battle. The dissipating brain fog, the diminishing fatigue, and the alleviation of joint pain and swelling offered glimpses of progress and promise.

As I navigated this journey of recovery, I was reminded of the importance of gratitude in the face of trials.

Despite the persistent challenges, I was filled with an overwhelming sense of thankfulness for the newfound relief and vitality that each day brought. Looking ahead, I was cognizant of the continued vigilance required in my recovery process. With continued annual eye scans as well as brain scans as needed and the prospect of ongoing blood thinner therapy, the road ahead remained uncertain yet hopeful.

In the darkness of fear and uncertainty, there always exists hope, a flicker that refuses to be extinguished. It is in these moments that we are called to summon the strength within us, transcend the limitations of our circumstances, and find solace in the power of ourselves. Each daunting challenge becomes an opportunity for growth, a chance to cultivate a mindset of unwavering determination and optimism.

———————

We may not be able to control the hand we are dealt, but we can choose how we respond to it. We can choose to embrace the uncertainty with courage and grace, to find beauty in the midst of chaos, and to discover strength in our vulnerability. In the face of overwhelming odds, we can find comfort in the knowledge that we are not alone and that there are others who have walked this path before us and who stand ready to offer support and solidarity. And so, we press on, guided by the belief that within every setback lies the seed of opportunity, and that within every challenge lies the potential for growth. For it is in the seasons of adversity that we discover the true measure of our strength, and emerge stronger, wiser, and more resilient than we ever thought possible.

10

JOY OF REMISSION

"I have told you these things so that you will be filled with my joy. Yes, your joy will overflow!"

— JOHN 15:11 (NLT)

L iving with a condition that is idiopathic, meaning it has no known cause, leads to much confusion on how to manage the symptoms. It feels as though every day is a guessing game as to what might or might not work and what might give relief or exacerbate symptoms. This is where I found myself post-surgery. I struggled at this moment to maintain a daily grasp on my positive mindset. I started to feel as though the balance that I was trying to achieve had become unachievable. Had the surgery truly been a success? If it had, then why did I feel so very awful and have new symptoms emerging on what felt like the daily? As much as I was ready to shed my dear friend Hank, it would seem we were meant to be lifelong partners.

Have any of you been to a place where your outer appearance does not match your inner turmoil? This is where I was beginning to find myself. In the midst of my ongoing battle with an incurable brain disease, I found myself navigating a delicate balance between appearance and reality. Despite the unseen struggles brewing within, the facade of wellness often earned me compliments on my appearance. I often heard things like, "You look so great; you must be feeling better." It's the curious paradox of this condition—the ability to maintain a facade of wellness despite the turmoil raging within. A touch of makeup and a positive attitude works wonders, casting a veil over the unseen battles being fought beneath the surface.

My primary focus at this point shifted to identifying and understanding my triggers, a crucial step in striving to achieve periods of remission.

As I struggled with the fluctuations of this relentless condition, I leaned into my journaling, seeking patterns within the chaos to decipher the elusive triggers behind the more intense symptoms that seemed to surprise me. Weather changes quickly became an apparent adversary to my condition, transforming me into an incredibly accurate human barometer. The shifting atmospheric pressures caused varying degrees of pain in my head and behind my eyes, a phenomenon that has led to intense joking that individuals with IIH should moonlight as meteorologists for their uncanny accuracy.

ACCEPTANCE, IT SEEMS, IS THE CORNERSTONE OF THIS JOURNEY.

While those of us living with IIH acknowledge that a life entirely free of symptoms may forever elude us, we must stay determined to carve out a path toward a more comfortable existence within the constraints of this unforgiving illness. The invaluable lesson I've gleaned from living with an incurable condition is the art of cherishing simple joys. Each good day is a treasure, sparking within me a childlike exuberance that defies the weight of my circumstances. I've come to embrace pain not as an enemy to be fought but as an insep-arable companion on this journey, a constant reminder of my unmatchable strength.

Through it all, I am learning the power of choice—the choice to maintain my sanity, to keep fighting, and to never surrender to despair.

Breakthroughs, I've come to realize, often emerge from the shadows of despair, reminding me that hope is a light that never truly fades. I've learned to release the burdens of the unchangeable, under-standing that all things, even pain, are transient. And so, I journey forward, not just one day at a time, but sometimes one precious moment at a time, armed with the unwavering belief that a good attitude can carry me through even the darkest of nights.

It was in one of these very darkest of nights that the blasting of light began to shine brightly for me. I had been going to a revival service at our church, just broken from the immense pressure of living under the burden of this condition for so very long. I found myself going back night after night, just wrought in emotions, praying for a moment of relief to regain the strength to fight for my life again.

On night three, as I sat at the back of the church auditorium, I remember praying for a glimmer of hope to light my way and give me strength to push forward. I went home that night and laid my head on my pillow, something that in nights past was the most dreaded part of my day, always being met with the ringing in my ears even louder. This night was different. I laid my head on my pillow, then lifted my head. I repeated this over and over to be sure, but the ringing in my ears was gone. What was this strange silence I was enjoying for the first time in forever?

With what appeared to be the elimination of my symptoms, I sched-uled an appointment with my eye specialist, Dr. Bloom. I braced myself for the too-familiar ritual of examinations and assessments.

As he meticulously reviewed my test results, a sense of anticipation hung heavy in the air, mingling with the faint echoes of past battles fought and endured. When Dr. Bloom entered the room, his demeanor reflected a hint of astonishment, a glimmer of something extraordinary brewing beneath the surface. "How are you feeling?" Dr. Bloom inquired, his voice tinged with a mix of curiosity and disbelief.

Gathering my thoughts, I mustered the courage to articulate the impossible. "I currently have zero symptoms." The words hung in the air, with the weight of disbelief and wonder.

Dr. Bloom's expression softened, a look of disbelief covering his face. "I don't know what to tell you, except I see no signs of distress in your eyes." He went on to explain how my optic nerves not only had stopped declining but had reversed and were not showing intense swelling as they had in exams past.

His words reverberated through the confines of the room, resonating with a depth of meaning that transcended the limits of language. Not only had my symptoms vanished, but the tests bore witness to a miraculous transformation. The damage once inflicted upon my body had been reversed, the scars of battle fading into oblivion. My optic nerves, once a battleground of affliction, now stood as a sign of health and vitality. In that moment, I stood on the precipice of disbelief and wonder, my faith emboldened by the undeniable evidence of divine intervention to bring my first remission.

As the reality of my miraculous remission washed over me, a surge of gratitude swelled within my soul.

"Don't you tell me my God can't do it!" I proclaimed, the words ringing with a resolute defiance against doubt and despair. For in that sacred moment, I bore witness to the boundless power of faith and the unfathomable depths of divine love. It was at this moment I felt such an overwhelming gratitude to those who had walked alongside me on this journey, who have offered prayers and solace in times of trial. I remember vividly just wanting to sit in this moment and soak it all in. I felt a wide range of emotions, from joy to anxiety. I was so filled with joy at the relief from symptoms yet anxious, not knowing for how long the relief might last. In either outcome, whether a short season or a long reprieve, I knew I was blessed with this season and determined to make the most of it.

To those still weathering their own storms, I offer a glimpse of hope and encouragement. Keep praying. Keep pushing. Keep believing. For even in the midst of the darkest moment, miracles await, positioned to unfold in the fullness of time. Stand firm in faith, for your miracle may be on the verge of arriving. Do not lose heart, for in the middle of adversity lies the promise of hope and renewal.

QUESTIONS FOR REFLECTION

Think about a moment in your journey that provided relief. Write that moment down and explain in detail how you felt.

Who is someone you can depend on while dealing with your chronic illness? Take a moment to write a note and tell them thank you for their support. It can become easy when living in daily pain to forget the support that we have around us.

Write down three positive words about yourself. These words you can take and write in areas of your home that you see frequently. They need to be there to remind you how strong you are and how able you are to keep fighting when the days get hard.

PART THREE
NAVIGATING CHALLENGES: DISCOVERING THE ART OF MODERATION

II

FROM REMISSION TO RELAPSE: DEALING WITH DEPRESSION AND ANGER

"The LORD is close to the brokenhearted; he rescues those whose spirits are crushed."

— PSALM 34:18 (NLT)

Well, well, well... Look who decided to drop by for a visit. It's none other than our old friend, Hank. You know, the unpredictable guest who never quite knows when to leave or to stay gone? Now, Hank's not exactly known for sending out formal requests before crashing into my life, but here we are again, facing the ebb and flow of this roller-coaster ride together. With the return of Hank came an emotional whirlpool—from the calm waters of remission to the stormy seas of relapse. I was left to navigate the murky depths of depression and anger.

I found myself standing at the threshold of acceptance, reluctantly welcoming Hank back into my life. But let's be real here—acceptance doesn't always come easy, especially when it's accompanied by a barrage of conflicting emotions. At this moment, I was knee-deep in the messy middle of grieving a new loss, and I'll admit, I was not handling it with grace. The facade of acceptance cracked, giving way to a flood of anger, tears, and every other emotion under the sun. And you know what? That's okay. Because sometimes, before we can rise, we need to allow ourselves to fall apart.

In the ever-changing landscape of living with IIH, the journey from remission to relapse can feel like sailing through unpredictable seas.

Just when you think you've found solid ground, the tides of relapse can sweep you back into the depths of uncertainty. However, it's not just the physical symptoms that accompany this rollercoaster; it's the emotional turbulence that often proves just as challenging to navigate.

I REMEMBER THAT FIRST WEEK AFTER MY RELAPSE, TEARS STAINED MY PILLOW AS MY EMOTIONS FLOODED MY EYES.

I entered my first day back to work, reliving all my symptoms with a hint of reluctance. As a piano teacher, I'm expected to uphold a face of strength throughout the day, delivering lessons with unwavering enthusiasm while concealing the turmoil raging within. The mothers who wait and listen during lessons often observe and mention my vibrant energy week after week, yet they are oblivious to the silent battle I wage inside. If only they knew the truth.

The week of my relapse, I remember enduring an arduous ten-hour workday; I concealed the excruciating pain pulsating behind my right eye, the telltale sign of spinal fluid seeping from its corner. Each minute of the day was a testament to my inner strength to endure as the crackling agony worked its way from my head to my feet. Movement became a cruel reminder of the fluid imbalance wreaking havoc within, tormenting every vertebra with its absence.

Despite the relentless grip and daily reminder of pain, Hank's presence still manages to catch me off guard at times. It was time for the spring performance in my studio. I had a grueling fourteen hours of setup, performance, and teardown, including the arduous task of moving the piano twice in the same day. The toll on my legs and feet was undeniable. Swelling, bruising, and excruciating pain served as stark reminders of the ongoing battle within me. Monday morning, I found myself crawling up the stairs of my own home, a humbling testament to the physical aftermath of my efforts. Yet, even amid this adversity, I found solace in the opportunity to rest briefly before embarking on another round of teaching later that day.

You may wonder, why subject myself to such strain? Simply put, Hank will not dictate the course of my life.

Teaching is my passion, and my students are my priority. The elaborate performances I orchestrate are not merely grand gestures, but heartfelt tributes to the dedication of my students throughout the year. Life's challenges may attempt to derail me, but for me, true strength is revealed in my response to adversity. This year, more than ever, has been a testament to that resilience.

In the face of my affliction, I have remained steadfast in my commitment to my students, consistently giving my all each and every week. My condition will never serve as an excuse to falter in my responsibilities. Should the day come when it impedes my ability to fulfill my duties, I will gracefully step away from teaching. For now, my mantra remains unwavering: pain may be temporary, even if temporary means the entirety of my earthly journey.

With the rise of all my old symptoms emerging, I made an appointment with my neurosurgeon for another scan to search for answers. All I could hold on to was the promise of answers, or perhaps even a glimmer of relief. As I prepared for my appointment, I glanced in the mirror to see my face swollen, distorted by the fluid cascading unchecked from my brain, rendering even the simplest movements agonizing. Smiling was becoming a challenge not only because of the emotional distress of my current situation but also due to the twitching of my facial muscles. I became plagued by relentless questions. Why was the stent not doing its job? Why did I experience such sweet relief to only be plagued by such a fierce storm so soon after? It's not a matter of fairness—life rarely is—but on days like this, I was missing the simplicity of days gone by. I longed to reclaim the life I had experienced even for a brief season, untainted by the shadow of Hank's relentless grip.

IN THE MIDST OF A RELAPSE, WRESTLING WITH DEPRESSION AND ANGER BECOMES A FORMIDABLE CHALLENGE.

It's crucial to acknowledge and accept these emotions as valid responses to the hardships endured. Seeking support from friends, family, or a support group can provide solace and understanding during these tumultuous times. Professional help from a therapist or counselor specializing in chronic illness can also offer invaluable guidance in navigating these complex emotions.

> On a more practical level, practicing self-compassion and prioritizing self-care are essential aspects of managing depression and anger.

Engaging in activities that bring comfort and joy, setting realistic expectations, and focusing on what can be controlled are vital strategies. It can become easy to sink into depression if anger is left unchecked for too long. Expressing those strong emotions through journaling can aid in processing feelings and finding relief. There is something healthy and even healing in putting your feelings down on paper. It provides a safe space for emotional expression, allowing you to articulate and process your complex feelings.

During a relapse, navigating through the tumultuous waves of depression and anger can feel like traversing a stormy sea with no end in sight. Another lifeline crucial for weathering the storm is connections with supportive friends and family. Having people surrounding you who will stand for you when you cannot find the strength to do so yourself is critical in overcoming the depression and anger a relapse can bring.

In the depths of despair, it's easy to fall prey to the overwhelming weight of negative emotions. Yet, holding on to hope becomes a life-line, a flicker of light that illuminates the path forward. It's a reminder that despite the current darkness, better days lie ahead. This brings hope that through the darkest nights, we can be reminded the storms eventually pass, making way for brighter horizons. In the face of relapse, it's not just about surviving but about persevering—holding on to the belief that even in the darkest moments, there exists the potential for growth, healing, and renewal. It's about embracing the journey with courage, resilience, and an unwavering determination to emerge from the shadows into the warmth of the sun once more.

12

UNCOVERING THE RISK OF SUICIDE: TAKING CONTROL OF YOUR THOUGHTS

"For I know the plans I have for you," says the LORD. "They are plans for good and not for disaster, to give you a future and a hope."

— JEREMIAH 29:11 (NLT)

In the depths of my journey with IIH, there's a shadowy path I've walked, one where the weight of my condition has pressed down on my spirit. It's a place where pain isn't just physical—it gnaws at the edges of my mind, threatening to consume me. There have been moments when the relentless headaches, the blurred vision, and the constant battle against fatigue felt like an endless storm raging within.

In those moments, it's not just my body that's weary; it's my soul. The relentless struggle, the uncertainty of what each day will bring, becomes too much to carry. And in those moments of despair, when hope seems like a distant memory, the thought of escape whispers its dangerous allure. Living with IIH is a daily fight—a fight against pain, against fear, against the overwhelming sense of isolation that creeps in when others can't understand the invisible battles I face.

It's easy to feel like I'm drowning in the depths of my own suffering like there's no way out.

I TYPICALLY PRIDE MYSELF ON BEING A VERY POSITIVE PERSON.

Someone who can take on every challenge head-on without fear of what the future might bring. So, imagine my surprise when the overwhelming emotions of life had a season of taking me over. As tears flowed down my cheeks, I stood at the kitchen counter, attempting to prepare lunch for my family. Unable to contain the weight of my emotions any longer, I turned to my husband, voice quivering, and confessed, "I don't think I can do this any longer. I don't think I can wake up tomorrow and face another day like this." The words hung in the air, heavy with the rawness of my feelings, a depth I hadn't yet revealed in my journey with IIH.

Sensing my distress, my husband abandoned his own tasks and approached, his concern evident in his eyes. "Hey, it's okay," he said softly, placing a comforting hand on my shoulder. "You don't have to apologize. What's going on? You know you can talk to me."

I wiped away tears as I struggled to articulate the overwhelming thoughts and emotions swirling inside my mind. "I know, I know, it's just... I feel like I'm drowning in this illness sometimes. Every day is a struggle and today... today just feels like too much."

I remember my husband's expression softened. I don't think he knew what exactly to say, but he wrapped his arms around me for a warm hug. "I understand," he whispered, his voice filled with empathy. "It's been a tough journey, and it's okay to feel overwhelmed sometimes. But remember, you're not alone in this. We're in this together, and we'll find a way through it."

In my whirlwind of emotions, I responded barely above a whisper, "I know, but it's just so hard to see any light at the end of the tunnel right now. I'm tired, physically and emotionally. I don't know if I have the strength to keep going."

My husband squeezed my hand gently, his eyes reflecting a quiet determination.

"You're stronger than you think, sweetheart," he reassured. "And it's okay to feel tired and scared sometimes. But we'll take it one day at a time, together. And we'll keep fighting, because I believe in you."

His unwavering support in this moment will stay with me in my memory. It was a crucial catalyst helping me through my darkest low.

I HAD TO FIGHT AND DIG TO RECLAIM MY LIFE FROM THAT POINT.

Life felt pointless, devoid of emotion, devoid of purpose. It was as though I was merely a spectator to my own existence, watching from a distance as the days passed by in a haze of indifference. In those moments, I felt like a shell of myself, stripped bare of the joy and vitality that once defined me. I trudged through each day with a heavy heart, the weight of emptiness pressing down on my soul. There were no highs, no lows—just a numbing sense of apathy that engulfed me entirely.

It was a lonely place to be, lost in the vast expanse of my own mind, disconnected from the world around me. I longed to feel something—anything—but the numbness persisted, an impenetrable barrier between me and the outside world. I've learned that even in the darkest moments, there's a flicker of light, a glimmer of hope that refuses to be extinguished. It's the warmth of a supportive friend, the comforting embrace of a loved one, the reassuring words of a healthcare provider who understands. It's the realization that you're not alone in this journey, that there are others who have walked this path before you and emerged stronger on the other side.

To you, my dear reader, who may find yourself grappling with the overwhelming weight of suicidal thoughts, I want you to know that you are not alone. In this moment of darkness, I extend my hand to you, offering a glimmer of hope in the midst of the shadows that threaten to engulf you.

First and foremost, please know that your life is precious, and your presence in this world is invaluable. You are worthy of love, of support, of compassion, and there are people who care deeply about you, even if it may not feel like it right now.

If you're struggling with suicidal thoughts, I urge you to reach out for help. It's okay to not be okay, and it's okay to ask for support. Talk to someone you trust—a friend, a family member, a counselor, a healthcare provider—anyone who can offer a listening ear and a shoulder to lean on. You don't have to carry this burden alone.

If you're in immediate danger or crisis, please seek help right away. Call emergency services, go to the nearest hospital emergency room, or reach out to a crisis hotline. Your safety is crucial, and there are trained professionals available 24/7 to provide the assistance you need.

Remember that suicidal thoughts are not a reflection of your worth as a person, but rather a sign that you're in pain and need support. Healing is possible, and there is hope for a brighter tomorrow. Take each day one step at a time, and be gentle with yourself as you navigate through this difficult time.

You are stronger than you know, and with the right support and resources, you can overcome this darkness and find light once again. Hold on to hope, my friend, and know that brighter days are ahead. You are loved. You are valued. You are not alone on this journey.

Cling to the moments of joy, however fleeting they may be, knowing that they are worth fighting for. Remind yourself that you are more than your illness! Repeat this after me—I am resilient, I am strong, and I am worthy of love and support. So, take each day as it comes, knowing that even in the midst of the storm, there is hope for a brighter tomorrow.

I WANT TO ENCOURAGE YOU WITH A MESSAGE OF HOPE.

While the journey through the depths of despair may seem endless, there are moments of joy waiting to be discovered, even in the lowest of places. Finding joy in the pain is not about ignoring or minimizing the struggles you face. Rather, it's about embracing the small moments of beauty, the fleeting glimpses of light that pierce through the darkness.

In your low place, I encourage you to seek out the things that bring you comfort and solace—the warmth of a cozy blanket, the soothing melody of your favorite song, the gentle touch of a loved one's hand. Allow yourself to savor these simple pleasures, to bask in the warmth of their embrace. Connect with nature, if you can. Spend time outdoors, breathing in the fresh air, feeling the sun on your skin, and marveling at the beauty of the world around you. Nature has a way of soothing the soul, of reminding us of the awe-inspiring miracle of life.

Engage in activities that nourish your spirit and bring you a sense of fulfillment. Whether it's painting, writing, gardening, or simply curling up with a good book, find something that speaks to your soul and allows you to express yourself authentically. And most importantly, surround yourself with love and support. Lean on your friends, your family, your community—those who lift you up and remind you of your worth. Share your struggles openly and honestly, and allow yourself to receive the compassion and understanding you deserve.

As you navigate the journey through the darkness, may you hold fast to the promise of brighter days ahead. May you find solace in the beauty that surrounds you and strength in the love that sustains you. And may you never lose sight of the hope that whispers softly in the quiet moments, reminding you that joy is always within reach, even in your lowest place.

13

JUGGLING RESPONSIBILITIES AND SELF-CARE

"You will keep in perfect peace all who trust in you, all whose thoughts are fixed on you!"

— ISAIAH 26:3 (NLT)

I wear many hats in life as most people do—I'm a devoted mother, a loving wife, a loyal friend, and a passionate business owner. Each role brings its own joys and challenges, but one thing remains constant: my tendency to put everyone else's needs before my own. From the moment I wake up in the morning, I'm on the go. There are lessons to plan and teach, emails to answer, meals to cook, and endless tasks to tackle. I move through my day with determination, always striving to be there for others in any way I can.

As a mother, my children are my top priority. I pour my heart and soul into raising them, nurturing their dreams, and supporting them through life's ups and downs. Their happiness and well-being mean everything to me, and I'll do whatever it takes to ensure they have the best possible start in life.

As a wife, I'm committed to supporting my husband and nurturing our relationship. We navigate life's challenges together, leaning on each other for support and strength. Living with a chronic illness has presented its own set of struggles and challenges for our marriage to tackle. Our love is the foundation that holds our family together, and I cherish every moment we share.

As a friend, I'm always there for those I care about, ready to offer a listening ear or a helping hand whenever it's needed. My friends know they can count on me, no matter what, and I take pride in being someone they can rely on. I love being able to cook a meal for someone, take a self-care gift to a pregnant friend, or send an encouraging note to someone struggling.

I am passionate about my work and dedicated to delivering the best possible service to my students and their families. I pour my heart and soul into every lesson, striving for excellence in everything I do. It is my desire to create a space for the students to learn, thrive, and excel. I work tirelessly to create exciting performance opportunities while supporting local businesses in my community. I attempt to make every family in the studio feel as though they are part of my family.

BUT AMID THE HUSTLE AND BUSTLE OF DAILY LIFE, I OFTEN FORGET TO PRIORITIZE MY OWN NEEDS.

I'm so busy taking care of everyone else that I neglect to take care of myself. I push myself to the limit, ignoring the signs of burnout and exhaustion until it's too late. It's a pattern I've fallen into time and time again—a pattern of self-sacrifice and neglect that leaves me feeling depleted and drained. But deep down, I know that I cannot continue down this path indefinitely. I know that in order to be the best mother, wife, friend, and business owner I can be, I need to prioritize my own well-being.

At times I feel as though I push so hard because living with a chronic illness has created a sense of pressure to do more and rest less, as if those of us living under a daily illness need to prove something to ourselves or others. It's like we feel the need to compensate for our illness by pushing ourselves beyond our limits, just to show that we're not defined by our condition. Our worth isn't measured by how much we can accomplish or how little we rest. It's okay to acknowledge our limitations and to prioritize our health and well-being above all else.

Living with a chronic illness is challenging enough as it is. We don't need to add extra pressure on ourselves to constantly prove our worth or capabilities.

It's important to remember that our value lies in who we are as individuals, not in what we can do or achieve. So, let's give ourselves permission to rest when we need to, to take breaks when we're feeling overwhelmed, and to ask for help when we need it. Let's focus on taking care of ourselves, both physically and emotionally, and let go of the need to constantly prove ourselves to others.

It's okay to pace ourselves, to set realistic goals, and to celebrate even the smallest victories along the way. We don't have to do it all, and we certainly don't have to do it alone. Let's show ourselves the same compassion and understanding that we so readily offer to others and remember that our worth is inherent—it doesn't need to be proven.

And so, with a newfound sense of determination, I had to learn how to embark on a journey of self-discovery and self-care. You might find yourself in a place of needing to take the time to do this as well. I had to learn how to set boundaries, say no when I needed to, and ask for help when I needed it.

If I am being perfectly honest here, I am still struggling with this. As a people pleaser, it is terribly painful to find time to put myself first or to say no to loved ones who depend on me. However, I am attempting to carve out time in my busy schedule for activities that nourish my soul—a weekend camping, a quiet cup of coffee while watching the sunrise, or sitting outside being amused by my small coop of chickens. Oh, the stories I have told my chickie girls that the world may never hear. They make for the best listeners, along with the finest of comic relief on a hard day.

Sitting cross-legged in the lush green grass of my backyard, I like to bask in the gentle warmth of the sun kissing my face. With closed eyes, I let the tranquil breeze weave through my hair, mingling with the soft, rhythmic clucks of my beloved chickie girls. Each cluck seems to carry a message of contentment and peace, as if the chickens themselves are joining in nature's symphony of serenity. It is in moments like this that I feel surrounded by the simple beauty of nature and the companionship of my feathered friends—a sense of calm washes over me, grounding me in the present and soothing the turbulence of my thoughts. Time seems to slow as I immerse myself in the tranquility of this idyllic scene, finding solace and rejuvenation in the harmonious balance of sun, breeze, and the gentle chatter of my flock.

You don't need to rush out and buy a flock of chickens to experience the kind of peace I've found in my backyard haven. What's essential is finding something, anything, that can distract your thoughts and bring you solace when your mind feels like it's spinning out of control. It could be a quiet moment in a sunlit corner of your garden, the soothing embrace of a favorite book, or even just a few minutes of deep breathing. Whatever it is, allow yourself the gift of that moment of calm within life's chaos. Trust me, it's worth it.

Slowly but surely, I am beginning to find balance in my life.

I am learning to give myself the same love and compassion that I so freely give to others. And in doing so, I have discovered a newfound sense of joy, fulfillment, and peace that I never knew was possible. As I look back on my journey, I realize that self-care isn't selfish—it's essential. It's what allows me to show up fully for myself and for those I love. And so, I encourage you to consider taking some time, even today, to prioritize your own well-being, knowing that in doing so, you're not only honoring yourself but setting an example for your children, husband, friends, and those around you.

For me, and maybe for you as well, the journey toward self-care is ongoing—a daily practice of love, acceptance, and forgiveness. But with each step I take, I'm reminded of the incredible power that lies within me—the power to create a life filled with joy, abundance, and infinite possibility, even in the face of living with chronic illness.

14

THE POWER OF NOT RIGHT NOW

"So be strong and courageous! Do not be afraid and do not
panic before them. For the LORD your God will personally
go ahead of you. He will neither fail you nor abandon
you."

— DEUTERONOMY 31:6 (NLT)

In the business of life, where the strain of responsibilities and obligations crescendos into a deafening roar, the concept of "not right now" emerges as a quiet yet potent refrain—a counterpoint to the relentless tempo of our daily routines. It's a subtle invitation to pause amid the chaos, to tune in to the rhythm of our bodies and minds, and to honor the wisdom that is within us.

In a culture that prizes productivity above all else, the notion of taking a step back can feel counterintuitive, even taboo. We're conditioned to push through discomfort, to soldier on regardless of the toll it takes on our physical, mental, and emotional well-being. Yet, in our relentless pursuit of achievement and success, we often overlook the vital importance of rest and recuperation.

What if we dared to challenge this paradigm? What if we acknowledged that our bodies are not machines, but living, breathing vessels that require nourishment, nurture, and restoration?

What if we recognized that by saying "not right now," we're not admitting defeat, but rather reclaiming agency over our lives?

In embracing the power of "not right now," we grant ourselves permission to set boundaries, to honor our limitations, and to prioritize our needs without guilt or shame. It's an act of self-care—an affirmation of our inherent worth and a testament to our commitment to living authentically, even in the face of societal pressure to do otherwise.

FEAR OF MISSING OUT

There are plenty of reasons we face, though, as to why we might choose not to say no. Let's unpack the pervasive fear of missing out (FOMO) that often looms large in the lives of those navigating chronic illness. Living with a condition like IIH and other chronic illnesses can already be isolating, with its demands and limitations distancing individuals from typical social engagements and activities. This sense of isolation can amplify the fear of missing out on opportunities for connection, experiences, and even career advancement. Consequently, the thought of declining invitations or requests can trigger anxiety about further detachment from the world outside of our illness.

FEELINGS OF GUILT

In addition to FOMO, coping with feelings of guilt when contemplating setting boundaries is a very real struggle. Despite facing significant physical and emotional challenges, we often face an internalized pressure to maintain a facade of normalcy and accommodate others' needs and expectations. This guilt can stem from a variety of sources, including societal norms, familial expectations, and personal standards of productivity and usefulness. As a result, the act of saying no can evoke feelings of selfishness or failure, compounding the already burdensome weight of chronic illness.

PEOPLE PLEASING

If having FOMO and guilt were not enough, we also like to sprinkle people pleasing into the mix. Many of us feel a deep pressure to please others and maintain relationships, which can pose a considerable obstacle to boundary-setting. Whether it's the fear of disappointing loved ones, the desire to avoid conflict, or the need to preserve a sense of belonging, we tend to find ourselves sacrificing our own well-being to prioritize the comfort and happiness of others. This external pressure can make it challenging to assert our needs and limitations, leading to a cycle of overcommitment and burnout.

FEAR OF PERCEPTION OF LAZINESS

I cannot tell you the number of times I have pushed through my day in immense pain simply because I did not want my family to perceive me as lazy. I will lay down on the couch for a few moments, then a sense of guilt rushes over me, and I am up again cooking, picking up, or cleaning because the last thing I want my friends and family to think is I am using my illness as an excuse for doing nothing.

The stigma surrounding chronic illness often fuels the fear of being perceived as lazy, unreliable, or exaggerating your condition. In a society that values productivity and self-sufficiency, we tend to struggle with needing validation and lack advocating for our own needs. The fear of judgment and misunderstanding can often deter us from asserting boundaries or disclosing the true extent of our health challenges, perpetuating feelings of isolation and alienation.

Navigating the complexities of boundary-setting is further complicated by the inherent challenges of managing a chronic health condition. From fluctuating symptoms and unpredictable flare-ups to the relentless demands of treatment regimens and medical appointments, we face a multitude of obstacles in prioritizing our own well-being.

This constant juggling act can make it difficult to establish and maintain healthy boundaries, leaving us feeling overwhelmed and depleted.

The persistent hope for improvement often leads us to say yes, clinging to the belief that pushing through the pain and fatigue will eventually yield a return to normalcy. This optimism, while understandable, can perpetuate a cycle of overcommitment and self-neglect, delaying the acceptance of our limitations and the implementation of effective boundary-setting strategies.

The lack of understanding from others about the true extent of the illness exacerbates these challenges, making it harder for individuals to assert their needs without fear of judgment or dismissal. Whether it's due to misconceptions about the severity of the condition, skepticism about invisible symptoms, or simply a lack of awareness and empathy, the lack of validation and support from friends, family, and even healthcare providers can leave us feeling invalidated and alone in our struggles. In light of these multifaceted challenges, it becomes increasingly evident that cultivating self-compassion, assertiveness, and clear communication is essential in navigating the complexities of boundary-setting while living with something like IIH.

LIVING WITH A CHRONIC ILLNESS IS LIKE NAVIGATING A CONSTANT BALANCING ACT, ISN'T IT?

It's this delicate dance between wanting to say yes to everything life throws at us and knowing when to put our foot down and say no.

Trust me, I get it—I've been there too. If I am being honest, I still struggle with this from time to time. It is a continual learning curve as we juggle life and living with a chronic illness. I have learned that setting boundaries and embracing the power of "not right now" is not just okay, it's essential for our well-being.

Here's the thing: saying yes to everything might feel like the right thing to do, especially when we're eager to prove ourselves or afraid of disappointing others. But the truth is, it's unsustainable.

It's like trying to pour from an empty cup—we can't give our best to others if we're running on fumes ourselves.

One particularly hectic weekend, I found myself juggling an overwhelming array of commitments without pausing to consider my own limits. I had my end-of-year piano performance, followed by officiating the wedding of an old piano student and then taking photographs of the happy couple afterward. As if that weren't enough, my son's eagerly anticipated fourth birthday party was also on the agenda for the following day.

With each event vying for my attention, I neglected to set boundaries or say no, fearing disappointing others more than I considered my own well-being. Despite the mounting exhaustion, I pushed through the first day, driven by a sense of obligation and determination. However, as the day drew to a close and I finally allowed myself a moment's rest, the toll of my relentless schedule became painfully apparent.

When I attempted to stand again, the sharp ache in my muscles made it clear I had pushed myself beyond my limits. I was in such immense pain that I was barely able to walk from the chair to my bed. The thought of facing another day of demands loomed dauntingly ahead. How would I summon the strength to celebrate my son's milestone birthday in the middle of my own physical depletion? It was a stark reminder of the consequences of setting unrealistic expectations and failing to prioritize myself—a lesson learned through painful experience.

So, how do we set boundaries and give ourselves permission to say, "Not right now"? It starts with tuning in to our bodies and listening to what they're telling us. Maybe it's that familiar pang of fatigue creeping in after a long day, or the subtle twinge of pain that's been lingering in the background. Whatever it is, honor it. Acknowledge that your body needs rest and that it's okay to take a step back.

But here's the tricky part: actually enforcing those boundaries. It can be tough, especially when we're worried about letting people down or missing out on opportunities. But remember, saying no isn't a sign of weakness—it's a sign of strength. It's about recognizing your limits and prioritizing your own well-being.

So, the next time you're faced with a decision, take a moment to pause and check in with yourself. Ask yourself, "Is this something I truly have the energy and capacity for right now?" If the answer is no, that's okay. It's not a reflection of your worth or your capabilities —it's simply a recognition of your current reality. Remember, setting boundaries isn't just about saying no—it's also about saying yes to yourself. It's about carving out time for the things that bring you joy, whether that's a leisurely stroll in the park, a cozy night in with a good book, or simply some much-needed alone time. Give yourself permission to set boundaries and embrace the power of "not right now." Your body will thank you for it, and so will your mind and soul.

15

LETTING GO OF EXPECTATIONS

"You can make many plans, but the LORD's purpose will prevail."

— PROVERBS 19:21 (NLT)

Ah, the art of letting go of expectations—a skill that seems as elusive as finding matching socks in a dryer. Picture this: You're sailing through the sea of life, map in hand, only to realize that your compass has gone rogue, and your ship has taken an unexpected detour through the Bermuda Triangle of expectations. How will we navigate the choppy waters of releasing the iron grip of expectations, both our own and those of others?

FROM THE EARLIEST DAYS OF MY CHILDHOOD, MY LIFE HAS BEEN METICULOUSLY PLANNED, EACH STEP CAREFULLY CRAFTED.

Even as a young child, I found solace in the structure of lists, enjoying the satisfaction of marking off each task, ensuring that nothing remained unfinished. From organizing my clothes by color and season to completing homework assignments with precision, I embraced the notion that a well-ordered existence was synonymous with success. This desire for planning permeated every aspect of my life, shaping my academic pursuits, career ambitions, and personal relationships. Whether charting out long-term goals or meticulously scheduling daily routines, I thrived on the sense of control and direction that planning provided.

However, despite my meticulous planning and unwavering dedication to order, life had other plans—ones that I never could have anticipated.

My old friend Hank waltzed into my life like an uninvited guest at a perfectly arranged dinner party. Hank has a knack for wreaking havoc on even the most carefully constructed plans, throwing curve-balls that leave me scrambling to catch my breath. Suddenly, the certainty I once clung to like a security blanket was replaced by gnawing uncertainty—a realization that each day held the potential for unforeseen challenges and disruptions. I can no longer rely on my trusty lists and schedules to navigate the unpredictable terrain of life with Hank by my side. Instead, I find myself grappling with a newfound sense of vulnerability, forced to relinquish control and embrace the uncertainty that Hank brings with him.

In life, we often find ourselves setting expectations for various reasons, each influenced by a combination of societal conditioning, personal desires, and cultural norms. From a young age, we accept societal expectations about success, happiness, and fulfillment from family, peers, and the media. These norms shape our aspirations and beliefs about what we should achieve in life. Setting expectations provides a sense of control and predictability in an uncertain world. By outlining goals and milestones, we feel empowered to shape our destinies and navigate life's challenges with purpose, all while staying in line with the mindset society has created for us.

When living with a chronic illness, the reliance on setting expectations can become a double-edged sword. On the one hand, it offers a sense of control and predictability in an otherwise unpredictable world of health fluctuations and uncertainties. By outlining goals and milestones, we can feel empowered to shape our future and navigate life's challenges with purpose, despite the limitations imposed by our condition.

HOWEVER, CHRONIC ILLNESS INTRODUCES A UNIQUE SET OF CHALLENGES THAT CAN DISRUPT THE FULFILLMENT OF OUR EXPECTATIONS.

Fluctuating symptoms, unpredictable flare-ups, and the need for ongoing medical management can throw even the most carefully crafted plans into disarray. If you happen to be a personality type like me, that likes structure, then this can lead to frustration, disappointment, and a sense of loss of control as we struggle to reconcile our expectations with the reality of our health condition. The pressure to meet societal or personal standards may exacerbate feelings of inadequacy and self-blame when chronic illness interferes with our ability to achieve set goals. The fear of falling short of expectations or being perceived as unreliable can further compound the emotional burden of living with a chronic illness.

Our own expectations often come from this fear of failure. Deep down, we are afraid we won't measure up to what society or even we ourselves think we should be.

We set the bar high as a way to protect ourselves from feeling let down or embarrassed. It's like we're always trying to prove ourselves, especially when we're dealing with a chronic illness. We want to show everyone we're still capable, still strong. We often pay a high price for this type of mindset.

Letting go of expectations, especially those we place on ourselves, can be a liberating journey toward inner peace and contentment. It's a process of self-discovery and self-compassion, where we learn to embrace each day as it comes, without the weight of unrealistic demands and pressures. It is important to acknowledge why we have these expectations in the first place. Once we recognize these expectations, the next step is to challenge them. Ask yourself: Are these expectations truly serving me, or are they hindering my growth and happiness? Be gentle with yourself as you navigate these questions. It's okay to let go of expectations that no longer align with who you are or who you want to become.

> One powerful practice in letting go of expectations is cultivating self-compassion. Treat yourself with the same kindness and understanding that you would offer to a dear friend.

Remind yourself that it's okay to make mistakes, to falter, and to not always meet every expectation perfectly. Allow yourself to be human, with all your flaws and imperfections. Living each day with grace means embracing the strength you have for that day, without forcing yourself to meet unrealistic standards. Some days, your strength might reveal itself as boundless energy and productivity, while other days, it might look like simply getting out of bed and taking care of yourself. It is important to understand that both days are perfectly okay.

Practice mindfulness to stay present in the moment, rather than getting lost in future expectations or past regrets. Focus on what you can control right now and let go of the rest. Trust in your ability to handle whatever comes your way, one step at a time. Surround yourself with a supportive community that uplifts and encourages you on your journey. Share your struggles and triumphs with others who understand and empathize with your experience. You will find in doing this that together, you can create a space where it's safe to let go of expectations and embrace the beauty of simply being yourself.

Letting go of expectations is not about lowering standards or settling for less. It's about freeing yourself from the shackles of perfectionism and embracing the fullness of who you are, with all your strengths and vulnerabilities. So be kind to yourself, dear reader, and allow yourself the grace to live each day to the fullest, in the strength you have for that day.

QUESTIONS FOR REFLECTION

Consider the concept of boundaries in relation to juggling responsibilities and self-care. Are there areas in your life where you struggle to set boundaries, leading to feelings of overwhelm or burnout? How might establishing clear boundaries benefit your overall mental health?

Reflect on the expectations you currently place on yourself. How do these expectations influence your thoughts, emotions, and behaviors? Are there any patterns or themes that stand out?

Reflect on a time when you experienced a relapse in your mental health journey. How did you navigate through it? What coping mechanisms or support systems did you find helpful during that time?

PART FOUR
LIVING WITH PURPOSE: BEFRIENDING HANK; NO LONGER ENEMIES

16

FROM STRUGGLE TO STRENGTH

"Dear brothers and sisters, when troubles of any kind come your way, consider it an opportunity for great joy. For you know that when your faith is tested, your endurance has a chance to grow. So let it grow, for when your endurance is fully developed, you will be perfect and complete, needing nothing."

–JAMES 1:2–4 (NLT)

Let's travel back a moment in the story to when Hank first entered my life. I remember the shock, the confusion, and yes, even the resentment that accompanied his arrival. Hank seemed like an unwelcome intruder, disrupting the rhythm of my life and challenging everything I thought I knew about myself. In those early days, I couldn't help but resent Hank for the havoc he wreaked on my body and mind. I resented the constant pain, the debilitating symptoms, and the limitations he imposed on my daily life. I resented the way he seemed to overshadow every aspect of my existence, leaving little room for anything else.

As time went on, I began to realize that resenting Hank was only making my journey more difficult. It was like carrying around a heavy burden, weighing me down and preventing me from moving forward. I knew that if I wanted to find peace and acceptance, I would need to change my perspective. So, slowly but surely, I began to shift my mindset. Instead of seeing Hank as an enemy to be defeated, I started to see him as a companion on my journey.

I have learned patience from Hank as I navigated through the uncertainties and setbacks of my journey. I have learned resilience as I faced each new obstacle with determination and courage. And perhaps most importantly, I learned acceptance—not just of Hank, but of myself and the journey I was on. It wasn't an easy process, by any means. There were moments of frustration, of anger, of despair. But through it all, I held on to the glimmer of hope that acceptance would eventually lead to peace. And you know what? It did. As I learned to embrace Hank as a part of who I am, I discovered a newfound sense of freedom. I no longer felt defined by my condition; instead, I felt empowered by it. Hank became not just a burden, but a badge of honor—a symbol of strength and resilience.

DO YOU FIND YOURSELF WONDERING WHERE TO GO FROM HERE?

If you find yourself fighting with feelings of resentment toward your own Hank, know that you are not alone. It's okay to feel angry, to feel frustrated, to feel overwhelmed. But don't let those feelings consume you. Instead, try to see Hank for what he truly is—a companion on your journey, guiding you toward greater understanding, acceptance, and ultimately, peace.

Maybe you are not at this point in your journey yet, so I hope to provide encouragement that your breakthrough in strength might be right around the corner. Each person's journey with IIH—with chronic illness in general—is unique, and there's no one-size-fits-all timeline for reaching acceptance. It's a process—a journey of self-discovery, growth, and healing. It is important to acknowledge and honor where you are right now. Give yourself permission to feel whatever it is you're feeling, without judgment or self-criticism.

As you navigate through these emotions, remember to be gentle with yourself. Healing takes time, and it's okay to take things one step at a time.

Allow yourself the space to grieve for the life you once had, while also embracing the possibilities of the life that lies ahead.

One helpful strategy on the road to acceptance is reframing your perspective. Instead of viewing your own Hank as an adversary, try to see him as a companion on your journey. Look for the lessons he has to offer, the opportunities for growth and self-discovery that lie hidden within the challenges he presents.

Seek out support from others who understand what you're going through. Whether it's friends, family members, support groups, or mental health professionals, surrounding yourself with a supportive community can make all the difference. Share your struggles and triumphs with others who can offer empathy, understanding, and encouragement along the way. Above all, remember that acceptance is not a destination; it's a journey—a continuous process of growth and self-discovery. Be patient and trust that you are exactly where you need to be at this moment. And know that no matter how long or challenging the road may seem, you are never alone.

THIS JOURNEY HAS LED ME FROM THE DEPTHS OF STRUGGLE TO THE EMPOWERING REALIZATION OF STRENGTH.

Living with IIH presents its own set of challenges, and at times, it's easy to feel defined by the diagnosis, to let it overshadow every aspect of our lives. But through this journey, I've come to understand that my identity is not confined to a medical label. I am more than my diagnosis. I am resilient. I am courageous. I am constantly evolving into the person I am meant to be.

In the journey of bringing this book to life, I've encountered a unique set of challenges stemming from my experience with IIH. Brain fog, alongside other symptoms, has often clouded my ability to articulate thoughts and ideas with clarity. On some days, the words flowed effortlessly onto the page, and I felt a sense of accomplishment in capturing the essence of my journey. Yet, there were also days when I found myself staring at a blank screen, grappling with a maze of jumbled words that refused to align.

Despite these hurdles, writing this book has become an integral part of my own narrative—a testament of the shift happening in my own life from struggle to strength.

It's been a journey of perseverance, as I've navigated through moments of frustration and exhaustion, digging deep to find the strength needed to continue. Through it all, I've learned to embrace the ebb and flow of the creative process, recognizing that each day brings its own unique challenges and opportunities.

We have to face things as more than just a task to check off a list, but more of a transformative journey of self-discovery and empowerment.

Consider this: What thoughts have been holding you back? What limiting beliefs have you internalized about your abilities and your future in the shadow of your chronic illness? It's time to challenge these narratives and recognize that your condition does not define you. Yes, living with a chronic illness presents unique challenges, but they need not dictate the trajectory of your life. It's about shifting your mindset from one of defeat to one of resilience, from viewing your struggles as insurmountable barriers to seeing them as catalysts for empowerment. It is a testament for all of us with chronic illness that the illness does not have to define our future or our abilities. It might take more effort and more time, but the end goal is still achievable.

ANOTHER IMPORTANT PIECE TO MOVING FROM STRUGGLE TO STRENGTH IS DISCOVERING YOUR IDENTITY BEYOND YOUR DIAGNOSIS.

This is not a task to be taken lightly, nor one that can be rushed. Instead, it requires a delicate balance of patience, time, and courage. At the outset of me trying to figure this out, I found myself confronted with the daunting task of letting go of preconceived notions. Preconceptions not only about who I thought I was supposed to be, but also about the limitations that my diagnosis imposed upon me.

For so long, my identity had been intertwined with my illness, as if it were an inseparable part of who I was. But as I began to peel back the layers, I realized that my illness did not define me; rather, it was just one aspect of my multifaceted identity.

With this realization came a newfound sense of freedom—a freedom to explore, to experiment, and to redefine myself on my own terms. Who is the new me? That question echoed in the recesses of my mind quite frequently. It took a long time for the answer to begin to reveal itself. I discovered that the new me was not defined by my illness, but rather by the qualities and attributes that made me unique. I unearthed hidden passions and interests that had long been overshadowed by the demands of my condition. I embraced my strengths—both those that had been forged in the fires of adversity and those that were dormant, waiting to be awakened.

Perhaps most importantly, I learned to embrace the complexities of my identity—the contradictions, the imperfections, and the moments of vulnerability that made me human. I found beauty in the messiness of life, in the interplay of light and shadow that danced across the canvas of my existence. This journey of self-discovery was not without its challenges. There were moments of doubt, moments of fear, and moments of uncertainty. Discovering my identity beyond my diagnosis was not just about finding answers; it was about asking the right questions. It was about peeling back the layers, confronting the shadows, and embracing the fullness of who I am.

I want to encourage you that you also have the power within you to redesign who you are in this new season of life. You are not bound by the constraints of a diagnosis. I encourage you to step boldly into this new chapter of your life, knowing that you have the power within you to create a life of meaning, fulfillment, and joy. Embrace the journey, trust in your resilience, and believe in the infinite possibilities that lie ahead. Your story is still being written; you hold the pen to author your own narrative. Rewrite the storyline from one constrained by an illness to one empowered because of an illness.

17

SETTING ACHIEVABLE GOALS

"We can make our plans, but the Lord determines our steps."

— PROVERBS 16:9 (NLT)

Navigating the terrain of setting achievable goals while living with a chronic illness is undoubtedly challenging. The balance between mental and physical abilities often feels like walking a tightrope, where one misstep can lead to setbacks and frustration. I, too, have found myself fighting with this struggle, feeling the weight of unmet expectations and the toll it takes on my well-being.

The key, I've come to realize, lies in finding a balance that honors both your mental and physical capabilities. It's about setting goals that are realistic and attainable, yet still challenging enough to inspire growth and progress. This requires a deep understanding of your own limitations, as well as a willingness to adapt and adjust as needed.

One strategy that has proven helpful for me is breaking down large goals into smaller, more manageable tasks. By focusing on bite-sized objectives, I'm able to make steady progress without overwhelming myself or exacerbating my symptoms. Additionally, I've learned to prioritize self-care and listen to my body, recognizing when it's time to rest and recharge rather than pushing myself beyond my limits.

Now, as I offer these insights, I speak not only as a guide but as a fellow traveler on this journey. I, too, recognize that I have much room to grow in this area. Despite understanding the importance of setting achievable goals and balancing mental and physical abilities, I still find myself struggling with the challenge of putting this knowledge into practice.

There are days when I feel invincible, bursting with energy and enthusiasm. On these days, the temptation to seize every opportunity and accomplish every task is overwhelming. I throw myself into each endeavor with fervor, determined to make the most of my newfound vitality.

Yet, in my eagerness to do it all, I often overlook the signs of fatigue and overexertion. Then, inevitably, the crash comes. The following days are a stark contrast to the euphoria of the previous ones. I find myself barely able to function, drained of energy and motivation. It's a humbling reminder of the limitations imposed by my chronic illness, a reminder of the need to set achievable goals. A reminder as well that I cannot continue to push myself beyond my limits without consequences. In these moments, I am reminded of the importance of pacing myself and listening to my body. It's a lesson I continue to learn, sometimes the hard way. I'm learning to recognize the signs of impending burnout and to honor my need for rest and rejuvenation.

> As I stumble and falter along the way, I'm committed to the journey of growth and self-discovery.

I know that progress is not always linear and that setbacks are an inevitable part of the process. Yet, with each stumble, I gain valuable insights and wisdom that guide me forward on my path. But perhaps most importantly, I've had to cultivate a sense of self-compassion and patience along the way. Living with a chronic illness means embracing the reality that some days will be better than others, and that's okay. It's about acknowledging the inherent unpredictability of the journey and learning to celebrate even the smallest victories.

SET ACHIEVABLE GOALS

Do you ever find yourself struggling to set achievable goals in the midst of your own journey with chronic illness? Know that you are not alone. It's okay to stumble, to falter, and to reassess your approach along the way. Remember to be gentle with yourself, to listen to your body, and to celebrate the progress you've made, no matter how small. And above all, know that you have the strength and resilience within you to overcome any obstacle that comes your way. We are not expected to be perfect. That is an unrealistic goal we tend to lay out for ourselves.

Setting achievable goals is a crucial aspect of personal development, especially for those of us living with chronic illness. It's imperative to approach goal setting with a structured method that takes into account the unique challenges and limitations imposed by health conditions. Begin by reflecting on your values and priorities in the context of your health. Understanding what matters most to you within the constraints of your condition provides a solid foundation for setting meaningful goals that contribute to your well-being.

Given the unpredictability of living with chronic illness, being specific in goal setting becomes even more vital. Define your objectives with clarity, considering how they align with your health needs and limitations. Whether it's managing symptoms, improving daily functioning, or enhancing overall quality of life, articulate your goals in a way that accounts for the realities of living with chronic illness.

Moreover, ensure your goals are measurable and realistic within the context of your health condition. Establish criteria for tracking progress that are sensitive to fluctuations in health status. Measurable goals allow you to monitor your achievements over time, providing motivation and a sense of accomplishment. Break down large goals into smaller, more manageable steps that accommodate the ebb and flow of your health.

Setting realistic goals is critical when living with chronic illness. Consider your current health status, treatment regimen, and energy levels when defining your objectives. While ambition is commendable, it's essential to set goals that are attainable given your health circumstances. Be mindful of pacing yourself and acknowledging the limitations imposed by your condition to prevent burnout and frustration.

SET FLEXIBLE DEADLINES

Setting deadlines can help maintain focus and momentum in pursuit of your goals. However, flexibility is key when navigating the challenges of chronic illness. Allow room for adjustments and modifications to your timeline as needed, taking into account fluctuations in health and energy levels.

Anticipate potential obstacles that may arise due to your health condition and develop strategies to overcome them. Seek support from healthcare providers, family members, or support groups who can offer guidance and encouragement. Collaboration and accountability can provide valuable resources for navigating the complexities of managing chronic illness while striving toward your goals.

Regularly monitor your progress and celebrate achievements, no matter how small. Recognizing and acknowledging milestones along the way reinforces your resilience and determination in the face of adversity. Setting achievable goals, especially while living with chronic illness, can feel like an uphill battle at times. But remember, every step forward, no matter how small, is a victory worth celebrating. Your journey is unique, and your resilience in the face of adversity is commendable. Keep moving forward, one step at a time, knowing that every step forward is progress, even if it is a small step.

CELEBRATE ACHIEVEMENTS

Celebrating achievements is a vital practice in maintaining self-encouragement while navigating life with IIH. In the face of constant challenges and setbacks, it's easy to become overwhelmed and discouraged. However, taking the time to acknowledge and celebrate our victories, no matter how minor they may seem, can be a powerful tool for bolstering our resilience and maintaining a positive mindset.

It is essential to redefine what constitutes an achievement. While traditional milestones like completing a project or reaching a goal are certainly worth celebrating, don't overlook the everyday victories that often go unnoticed. Perhaps it's getting out of bed on a particularly difficult morning, managing your symptoms effectively for a day, or even just finding a moment of peace amid the chaos of chronic illness. Each of these moments deserves recognition and celebration.

Make sure to establish rituals or practices that allow you to commemorate your achievements in a meaningful way. This could be as simple as journaling about your accomplishments, creating a gratitude list at the end of each day, or treating yourself to something special when you reach a significant milestone. The key is to find methods that resonate with you personally and make you feel acknowledged and appreciated for your efforts.

Don't hesitate to share your achievements with others. Whether it's confiding in a trusted friend or family member, joining a support group, or sharing your successes on social media, external validation can be incredibly affirming and motivating. You never know who you might inspire or uplift with your story. Remember to celebrate not only the outcome but also the journey itself. Life with chronic illness is learning to create a rhythm along the journey.

18

THE POWER OF CREATIVE OUTLETS

"For everything there is a season, a time for every activity under heaven."

— ECCLESIASTES 3:1 (NLT)

In the hustle and bustle of life, I found that the challenges that chronic illness continued to bring felt overwhelming most days. Days filled with medical appointments, treatments, and the constant struggle against the unknown can weigh heavy. I began searching for an outlet to let my thoughts escape. I discovered solace in various creative outlets scattered throughout my life—taking my children to paint pottery, escaping to nature to camp, letting the music take my mind to another place, letting my thoughts flow through writing, and playing a piano that echoed with melodies of possibility.

With hesitant hands, I delved into each medium, allowing my emotions to flow freely. Through the painting of clay, the calming sound of running water in the woods, and the gentle melodies of the piano keys, I found a refuge—a sanctuary where the weight of illness seemed to momentarily lift.

Engaging in activities like painting pottery with my children provided not just a distraction but a profound sense of connection and accomplishment. The tactile sensation of clay, the vibrant colors, and the shared joy of creation offered a sanctuary where the weight of illness momentarily lifted. Similarly, escaping to nature through camping became a source of solace. Surrounded by the tranquil beauty of the wilderness, away from the clamor of daily life, I found peace and perspective in the rustling of leaves and the vast expanse of the starry sky.

Music, too, emerged as a powerful ally in my journey. Playing the piano became a form of meditation, a mindful escape into the rhythmic flow of notes and the harmony of melodies. Each chord struck seemed to quiet the noise within, offering respite from the storm raging inside. Writing, meanwhile, became my therapy—a means of processing emotions and untangling the knots of thought that threatened to overwhelm me. Through journaling, I found clarity, transforming inner turmoil into tangible expressions of resilience and hope.

My creations became a reflection of my journey—a testament to resilience, faith, and hope.

Inspired by the transformative power of creativity, I reached out to others facing challenges of their own, inviting them to join me in exploring the healing potential of artistic expression. Together, we embraced a multitude of creative outlets. Through our collective efforts, we painted a new narrative—one filled with courage, compassion, and the unwavering belief that beauty can emerge from even the darkest of circumstances.

As I stood surrounded by my creative endeavors, I knew that each moment of artistic expression was not just a fleeting escape, but a strand of hope guiding me through the shadows of adversity. And in that realization, I found the courage to embrace the beauty of life, one creative endeavor at a time. In the midst of tumult, creative outlets are a powerful ally.

These aren't mere distractions, but lifelines, offering tangible relief and profound medical benefits. Picture yourself surrounded by loved ones, painting pottery in a cozy studio, or escaping to the tranquility of nature for a weekend camping trip. These moments aren't just about enjoyment—they're about stress reduction and pain management. Engaging in creative activities triggers the release of endorphins, your body's natural painkillers, providing a respite from the physical toll of chronic illness.

NOW, LET'S TALK ABOUT THE MENTAL LANDSCAPE.

As you delve into the world of creative expression, whether through music, writing, or visual arts, you're not just creating art—you're nourishing your mind and soul. The act of creation stimulates the production of neurotransmitters like dopamine and serotonin, lifting your mood and sharpening your cognitive function. Think of it as a workout for your brain, strengthening neural pathways and enhancing memory and problem-solving skills.

Here's where it gets even better: Creativity isn't just a solo endeavor. It's a bridge that connects you to others who share similar experiences.

Picture yourself in a room filled with fellow creatives, all navigating their own health journeys. Together, you share stories, swap tips, and find solace in the shared understanding of your struggles. This sense of community isn't just emotionally comforting—it can improve your overall well-being.

As you lose yourself in the flow of creative expression, whether it's strumming a guitar or getting lost in a novel you're writing, you're practicing mindfulness without even realizing it. You're fully immersed in the present moment, letting go of worries about the past and future. This state of mindfulness isn't just relaxing—it's transformative. It eases anxiety, reduces stress, and cultivates a deep sense of inner peace. As we navigate the challenges of chronic illness, we have to remember this: Creativity isn't just a luxury—it's a necessity. It's your secret weapon against the darkness. It brings joy to even the most difficult of days. So, pick up that paintbrush, strum that guitar, or open that journal. Let your creativity soar, and watch as it transforms not just your art but your entire outlook on life.

You might be thinking, "But I'm not a creative person. How can I tap into these benefits?" Well, here's the thing: Creativity isn't reserved for a select few. It's a fundamental aspect of being human, and everyone has the capacity to unlock their creative potential. So, if you've never explored creative outlets before, don't worry—you're not alone, and there are plenty of ways to dip your toes into the world of creativity.

You can start by considering your interests and hobbies. What activities bring you joy or pique your curiosity? Whether it's gardening, cooking, photography, or even rearranging furniture, there's creativity to be found in almost every pursuit. Start by experimenting with different activities to see what resonates with you.

Another approach is to step outside your comfort zone and try something entirely new. Take a painting class, join a community choir, or sign up for a writing workshop. Embrace the opportunity to learn and grow, and don't be afraid to make mistakes along the way. Remember, creativity thrives on exploration and experimentation.

If you're still unsure where to begin, consider seeking inspiration from the world around you. Take a walk in nature, visit an art gallery, or listen to music that moves you. Pay attention to the little moments of beauty and wonder that spark your imagination. You might be surprised by the creative ideas that emerge when you open yourself up to new experiences. Don't be too hard on yourself. Creativity is a journey, not a destination, and it's okay to start small.

Celebrate your successes, no matter how modest, and remember that every creative endeavor is an opportunity for growth and self-expression.

———————

Regardless of whether you've always considered yourself a "creative" person or are venturing into uncharted artistic territory, the benefits of engaging in creative outlets for managing chronic illness like IIH are undeniable. From stress reduction and pain management to enhanced mood and social connection, creativity offers a multifaceted approach to healing and resilience. As you embark on your journey of exploration and self-discovery, may you find solace, inspiration, and transformation in the boundless world of creative expression.

19

TOGETHER WE THRIVE

"So encourage each other and build each other up, just as you
are already doing."

— 1 THESSALONIANS 5:11 (NLT)

Amid the whirlwind of managing chronic illness, it's easy to overlook the profound impact of the support network that surrounds you. However, taking the time to reflect on your personal village—no matter how small—can be a transformative exercise in gratitude.

Let me speak to you from my heart, reader, about the profound importance of cultivating gratitude, especially in the context of living with IIH. You see, inside the turmoil of symptoms and treatments, it's all too easy to get lost in a sea of frustration and despair. Trust me, I've been there. The relentless nature of chronic illness can leave us feeling drained and disheartened, making it challenging to find reasons to be thankful.

But here's the thing: Even in the darkest of times, there are still blessings to be found, if we're willing to look for them. It's about shifting our perspective, from dwelling on what's going wrong to acknowledging what's still going right. It's about finding gratitude not only in the big moments of triumph but also in the small victories and everyday blessings that often go unnoticed.

BELIEVE ME, I KNOW IT'S NOT EASY.

There are days when the pain is so overwhelming, when it feels like there's no light at the end of the tunnel. But it's precisely in these moments that practicing gratitude becomes most transformative. I urge you to take the time to cultivate gratitude in your life, even when it feels like the hardest thing in the world. Trust me when I say that it's worth it. It's a reminder that no matter how tough things may seem, there is still beauty and goodness to be found in the world around us.

And in the end, it's gratitude that will sustain us, empower us, and light our way forward on this journey with IIH.

Gratitude can start by considering the individuals who have stood by you through thick and thin, offering unwavering support and companionship. It may be a close friend who has been a constant source of strength, listening to your worries and sharing in your triumphs without judgment. Or perhaps it's a family member whose love and care have been light during the darkest of times, providing comfort and reassurance when you needed it most.

Your village extends beyond just individuals—it may also include support groups or online communities where you find solace and understanding among others who share similar experiences. These spaces offer a sense of belonging and validation, allowing you to connect with others who truly understand the challenges you face.

Take a moment to reflect on the significance of these connections in your life. Consider the ways in which they have supported you, uplifted you, and helped you navigate the complexities of living with chronic illness. Recognize the strength and resilience that these relationships have instilled in you, empowering you to face each day with courage and determination.

Remember, your village doesn't have to be large to make a meaningful impact. Even one person who stands by your side with unwavering support can make all the difference. So, cherish these connections, nurture them, and express your gratitude to those who make up your personal village. For they are the ones who help you thrive, even in the face of adversity.

As I have reflected on my personal journey, I find myself overwhelmed with gratitude for the incredible village of people who have walked alongside me on this journey of navigating chronic illness. My village has stood by my side, offering unwavering love, support, and companionship through the trials and triumphs of life I have faced. In the depths of uncertainty and the times of adversity. Simply having support makes walking a tough road more bearable. The warmth of family, the comfort of friends, the camaraderie of support groups, and the expertise of a dedicated medical team have illuminated the path forward, infusing my days with hope, resilience, and an unwavering sense of belonging.

Living with a chronic illness can often feel like navigating through a lonely daily valley of pain and uncertainty.

In these moments, building a community of support becomes not just important, but essential. However, it's equally vital to remember that while we seek solace in our own villages, we must also strive to be that same supportive community for others. In the middle of our daily struggles and pain, it's easy to become consumed by our own challenges, but we mustn't forget that our friends, family, and fellow community members have their own trials and tribulations.

It is a truth as profound as it is challenging. Sometimes, when we're grappling with our own struggles, it can feel overwhelming to be there for others who are going through difficult times. Yet, in my own journey with IIH, I've come to realize that offering support to those we care about, even when we're struggling ourselves, is not only possible but also deeply rewarding.

REMEMBER, IT IS ESSENTIAL TO ACKNOWLEDGE AND HONOR OUR OWN LIMITATIONS.

It's okay to admit when we're feeling overwhelmed or drained. Taking the time to recharge and replenish your own reserves allows you to show up more fully and authentically for others. That being said, being there for someone in their time of need doesn't always require grand gestures or exhaustive efforts. Sometimes, it's the simple acts of listening, offering a shoulder to lean on, or just being present that make the biggest difference. Even if we can't offer solutions or fix their problems, our presence alone can provide comfort and solace.

You have to keep in perspective the importance of communicating openly and honestly with the person you're trying to support. Let them know that while you may be struggling yourself, you're still here for them, even if your capacity to help may be limited at times. Setting boundaries and managing expectations can help prevent feelings of resentment or burnout on your part while still allowing you to offer meaningful support.

As we lean on others for support, let us also extend a hand of compassion and understanding, recognizing that we are all on this journey together. By fostering a culture of mutual support and empathy, we create a stronger, more resilient community—one where we lift each other up, share our burdens, and thrive together despite the challenges we face.

20

WE ARE STRONG; WE ARE IIH WARRIORS

"Search for the LORD and for his strength; continually seek him."

— 1 CHRONICLES 16:11 (NLT)

On the battlefield of living with idiopathic intracranial hypertension, every day is a test of our resilience and fortitude. We wake up to a world where pain, uncertainty, and challenges loom large, yet we refuse to be defeated. Instead, we armor ourselves with courage, drawing strength from the depths of who we are to confront the obstacles that lie ahead. It's not just a matter of enduring the struggles; it's about embracing them as opportunities to showcase our unwavering determination.

As IIH warriors, we are bound together by a shared sense of purpose and camaraderie. In the face of adversity, we stand united, a formidable force that cannot be broken. Through our collective efforts, we transform moments of hardship into opportunities for growth and empowerment. We draw inspiration from each other's stories of courage, finding solace in the knowledge that we are not alone in our struggles.

AT THE HEART OF EVERY IIH WARRIOR LIES A RESERVOIR OF STRENGTH THAT KNOWS NO BOUNDS.

It is what propels us forward in the face of adversity, the courage that fuels our determination, and the unwavering resolve to never surrender to the challenges we face. Despite the pain, the uncertainty, and the setbacks, we draw upon this inner strength to navigate the complexities of living with IIH with grace and fortitude.

Our journey as IIH warriors is marked by both triumphs and tribulations. Each victory, no matter how small, is a testament to our strength. Whether it's managing symptoms, finding effective treatments, or simply getting through another day, we celebrate these milestones with unwavering pride and gratitude. When faced with setbacks or challenges, we refuse to be deterred. Instead, we rise to the occasion with renewed determination, ready to overcome whatever obstacles may come our way.

Perhaps the most remarkable aspect of our journey as IIH warriors is the sense of empowerment that comes from supporting one another.

In our community, every voice is heard, every story is valued, and every individual is embraced with empathy and compassion. Through our shared experiences, we not only find strength in solidarity but also inspire one another. In this nurturing environment, our shared experiences become the threads that weave together the fabric of our resilience.

Our community is not just a source of comfort—it's also a wellspring of inspiration. As we witness the courage and tenacity of our fellow warriors, we are reminded of the strength that lies within each of us. Their stories of perseverance ignite a fire within our souls, propelling us to reach new heights of bravery and determination. Through their triumphs, we find hope; through their resilience, we find strength.

We are more than just a collection of individuals—we're a force to be reckoned with. Together, we stand as living testaments to the power of solidarity, resilience, and compassion. As we continue on our journey as IIH warriors, we do so with the knowledge that we are stronger together, bound by the unbreakable ties of support that define us as a community.

Our community of IIH warriors is a tapestry woven from threads of diversity—diversity in experiences, backgrounds, and perspectives. Each of us brings a unique story to the table, shaped by our individual journeys with IIH. Some of us may have been diagnosed recently, while others have been battling this condition for years. Some of us are young, while others are older. Some of us are male, while others are female. Yet, despite these differences, we are united by a common bond—the shared experience of living with IIH. Our diversity is our strength, enriching our community with a wealth of insights, knowledge, and perspectives that enhance our collective understanding.

Advocacy lies at the very core of our identity as IIH warriors, serving as a potent tool for driving positive change and elevating the visibility of our condition within the broader healthcare landscape. It's not just about fighting for our own health and well-being; it's about paving the way for a better future for all those affected by IIH. Through our collective efforts, we strive to shine a spotlight on the challenges and barriers faced by individuals living with IIH, fostering greater understanding and empathy within our communities.

We may be rare, but we are an undeniably powerful force.

Our voices, though few in number, carry the weight of an entire community united in the pursuit of answers and solutions for our condition. We deserve not just to be heard, but to be listened to with earnest attention and urgency. It is only through amplifying our voices and advocating for the recognition and understanding of our unique challenges that we can pave the way toward advancements in the treatment and management of our condition.

Our advocacy extends beyond mere awareness-raising to encompass the pursuit of tangible improvements in access to healthcare resources and treatments for IIH. We recognize the critical importance of ensuring equitable access to timely diagnosis, comprehensive care, and innovative treatment options for all individuals living with IIH. By advocating for increased research funding, improved healthcare infrastructure, and enhanced support services, we strive to create a more supportive and inclusive environment for those navigating the challenges of IIH.

As we come together as a unified force, we empower ourselves and others to advocate for the resources and support needed to improve the lives of those living with IIH. Our advocacy efforts not only serve to elevate the voices of IIH warriors but also inspire hope, drive progress, and ultimately contribute to a brighter future for the entire IIH community. In essence, advocacy is not just a means to an end—it's a powerful expression of our collective strength, resilience, and unwavering commitment to making a meaningful difference in the lives of others.

"We Are Strong; We Are IIH Warriors" is a testament to the unbeatable spirit and unwavering determination that defines us as a community. Together, we stand as a light in a dark tunnel, ready to face whatever challenges may come our way. With courage in our hearts and strength in our souls, we march forward, united in our commitment to overcome adversity and reclaim our lives from the grip of IIH.

QUESTIONS FOR REFLECTION

How do you define inner strength, and how has your understanding of it evolved over time?

Reflect on a time when you received support from others during a challenging period in your life. How did it impact you?

What does it mean to you to be an IIH warrior, and how has your journey shaped your identity?

ACKNOWLEDGMENTS

Along my journey, I have been continually humbled by the overwhelming support I have received. I have friends who have consistently checked in on me to see how I am, both physically and mentally. There have been meals cooked and brought to my house, scripture sent with a prayer or an encouraging note, flowers left by my door, and on and on. My village of people has stretched from my close family to friends, studio parents, and support group connections.

As I reflect, one truth stands out above all: I am endlessly grateful for each and every person in my circle. To my family, whose unwavering love and support have been my anchor in the stormiest of seas, I owe an immeasurable debt of gratitude. Your presence, your understanding, and your unwavering belief in me have carried me through the darkest of days.

To my friends, whose laughter and companionship have brought light to even the heaviest of moments, thank you for standing by my side with unwavering loyalty and kindness. Your presence has been a balm to my soul, reminding me that I am never alone on this journey.

To the support groups and communities that have welcomed me with open arms, offering empathy, understanding, and a safe space to share my struggles, thank you for reminding me that there is strength in vulnerability and power in solidarity.

To my dedicated medical team, whose expertise, compassion, and unwavering commitment to my well-being have been a lifeline in the face of uncertainty, I am endlessly grateful. Your guidance and care have not only alleviated my physical symptoms but have also instilled in me a sense of hope and resilience that I carry with me each day.

In the tapestry of my life, each of you has woven a thread of love, support, and compassion that I cannot imagine my journey without. Together, we have weathered storms, celebrated victories, and forged bonds that are unbreakable. As I navigate the challenges of managing my condition, I find solace in knowing that I am surrounded by such a remarkable village of people who love me and my family and, more importantly, pray daily for me for strength and guidance. So, from the depths of my heart, I extend the largest thank you to my personal village of people—I truly do not know what I would do without you.

ABOUT THE AUTHOR

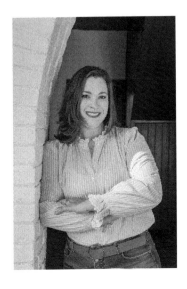

Bridgette Finley's life is a tapestry woven with threads of resilience, passion, and unwavering faith. At the heart of her narrative lies a deep commitment to faith, family, friends, music, nature, and the pursuit of knowledge—a journey colored by both triumphs and challenges.

As a devoted mother of three and a loving wife, Bridgette finds profound fulfillment in nurturing her family and sharing her love for music through her roles as a piano studio owner and teacher. Her piano studio remains a sanctuary where she shares her love for music, inspiring her students with her dedication and creativity.

Her children are the heartbeat of her life. Whatever her children are doing, she loves being right there beside them. From sitting for hours on end for dance practice to playing with chickens in the backyard to getting wrapped up in a heartfelt conversation. If her children are interested, she is an active part.

She also loves cooking. Having an open-door policy for family and friends, and strangers when needed, has always been the core of who Bridgette is. She loves to connect and encourage those in her life and around her community.

Bridgette's path took an unexpected turn with the diagnosis of IIH (Idiopathic Intracranial Hypertension). This condition introduced complexities and uncertainties into her life, challenging her to redefine resilience in the face of adversity. Despite its impact, Bridgette steadfastly refuses to let IIH define her. It is a part of her journey, not the destination.

For Bridgette, the bad days do not define the everyday. While IIH presents its challenges, it is just one thread in the rich tapestry of her existence—a thread that she confronts with courage and grace. Instead of succumbing to fear or self-pity, she has chosen to embrace each day with a determination to live fully and joyfully. Her fire and fight for life burn brightly, undeterred by the hurdles she faces.

Bridgette finds solace and inspiration in nature. Camping trips with her family offer moments of respite, grounding her in the beauty of creation and strengthening her resolve. Family camping trips become sanctuaries where she connects deeply with the beauty of God's creation, renewing her spirit and fostering cherished memories with her family.

Bridgette's story is not just about overcoming challenges; it's about embracing life fully and finding strength in vulnerability. Rooted in faith and guided by a relentless pursuit of growth, she continues to inspire others with her unwavering optimism and resilience. Her journey is proof of the unyielding belief that every obstacle is an opportunity for growth. Bridgette's life resonates with a melody of hope and courage—a symphony of grace that leaves an indelible mark on all who have the privilege of knowing her.

INVITE BRIDGETTE TO SPEAK

Bridgette would be honored to share her story with you as well as your organization, group, and community.

While she is happy to tailor her speaking engagement content to the needs of each audience and the goals of the event, her most requested speaking engagements include:

- **Personal Journey with IIH**: Insights into living with and managing IIH, based on her book, *Hank in My Head*.
- **Awareness and Advocacy**: Information on IIH to help raise awareness and foster understanding.
- **Q&A Sessions**: Interactive discussions to address specific questions and concerns about IIH.

To inquire about her availability and discuss details of your event, visit bridgettefinley.com and complete the Request to Book form. Bridgette will get back to you as soon as possible to discuss how she can collaborate with you to make your event a success.

APPENDIX
WRITTEN BY: DR. STUART YOUNG, OD, FCOVD

IDIOPATHIC INTRACRANIAL HYPERTENSION SYMPTOMS

- Headache: the most commonly reported symptom.
- Transient episodes of visual loss (usually lasting seconds): often following changes in posture.
- Pulsatile tinnitus: a unilateral "whooshing" sound exacerbated with positional changes. It is considered to be specific for the diagnosis.
- Visual disturbance: typically involves the peripheral visual field. Visual acuity (central vision) is not usually affected and is more a sign of advanced disease.
- Horizontal diplopia (double vision): occurs among patients with associated unilateral or bilateral non-localizing sixth cranial nerve palsy.

WHAT THE EYE DOCTOR WILL LOOK FOR

- A complete ocular examination, including a dilated fundus examination.
- Visual field examination.
- Optic nerve photographs.
- On initial presentation, neuroimaging is needed to exclude secondary causes of intracranial hypertension. Magnetic resonance imaging (MRI) and MR venography (MRV) of the brain are usually the imaging modalities.
- Follow-up appointments will be done at three months, six months, or twelve months, depending on symptoms of optic nerve appearance.

INFORMATION WAS TAKEN FROM

Review of Optometry: https://www.reviewofoptometry.com/article/ro1117-a-second-helping

The American Academy of Ophthalmology: https://eyewiki.org/Pseudotumor_Cerebri_(Idiopathic_Intracranial_Hypertension)

Made in the USA
Columbia, SC
06 March 2025

54738735R00087